THE NEW MEDITERRANEAN
DIET

EXTEND YOUR LIFE WITH THE BEST FOOD PROGRAM IN THE WORLD.
THE BASIC PRINCIPLES, THE NEW FOOD PYRAMID WITH THE FOODS TO BE PREFERRED FOR A HEALTHY AND FIT LIFE.

KELI BAY

The New Mediterranean Diet

CONTENTS

INTRODUCTION

Mediterranean diet is a specific diet by removing processed foods and high in saturated fats. It's not necessarily about losing weight, but rather a healthy lifestyle choice. It is about ingesting traditional Ingredients consumed by those who live in the Mediterranean basin for a long time. Their diets never changed, so they must be doing something right. This is a diet rich in fruits, vegetables, and fish. Cooking with olive oil is a fundamental ingredient and is an ideal replacement for saturated fats and Trans fats. Vegetables and fruits grow well in the heat of the Mediterranean continents, so it's not surprising that the locals devour plenty of them. Studies show that the people who live in these regions live longer and better lives. Changing your own eating habits to one that is proven to be healthy is a good enough reason to begin.

Many studies that have been done on the Mediterranean diet offered promising results.

Heart-healthy diet. Blood pressure tends to drop significantly on the Mediterranean diet; in other words, is a natural way to lower the risk of cardiovascular disease. Researchers have found that the Mediterranean diet can lower your chances of having a stroke and other vascular diseases.

Reduced risk of certain cancers. In general, the Mediterranean diet emphasizes eating plant-based foods and limiting red meat, bad oils, and processed foods. Hence, these eating habits may provide some protection against malignant diseases. People in Mediterranean countries are overall less likely to die from cancer.

Neuroprotective benefits. The Mediterranean diet may improve brain and cogitative functions in older adults (by 15 percent). Clinical trials have shown that those who followed this dietary regimen were less likely to develop Alzheimer's, dementia, or insomnia. A new study has found that antioxidants in the Mediterranean diet plan may protect brain and nerves, cutting the risk of neurological disorders by almost 50 percent.

Weight loss. The Mediterranean diet is the most natural and most delicious way to lose weight and maintain ideal body fat percentage. Low-calorie foods such as fruits, vegetables, yogurt, and fish are widely used in the countries that border the Mediterranean Sea. Natural appetite suppressants include beans, legumes, fat fish, plain dairy products, and high-fiber foods (almost all vegetables, whole grains, apples, avocado, and chia seeds). Ginger may control the hunger hormone "ghrelin" too. Consuming a small amount of honey has been shown to reduce appetite. And you will become one step closer to dropping serious pound!

Longevity. Basics of this dietary plan are however vital to longevity and healthy leaving. Other unexpected benefits include reduced risk of developing depression, diabetes management, improved gut health and better mood.

CHAPTER 1

THE NEW MEDITERRANEAN DIET: THE MOST RECENT EVOLUTION

Just like it sounds, the Mediterranean diet comes from the dietary traditions of the people of the Mediterranean isle region such as the Romans and Greeks. The people of these regions had a rich diet full of fruits, bread, wine, olive oil, nuts, and seafood. Despite the fatty elements in their diet, the people of this region tended to live longer and overall healthy lives with relatively less cardiovascular heart issues. This phenomenon was noticed by American scientist Ancel Keys in the 1950s.

Keys was an academic researcher at the University of Minnesota in the 1950s who researched healthy eating habits and how to reverse the decline in American cardiovascular health. He found in his research that poor people in the Mediterranean region of the world were healthier compared to the rich American population which had seen a recent rise in cardiovascular heart issues and obesity. Compared to wealthy New Yorkers, the lower class in the Mediterranean lived well into their 90s and tended to be physically active in their senior years. Keys and his team of scientists decided to travel the world and study the link between the region's diet and the health of the people who lived there. In 1957, he traveled and studied the lifestyles, nutrition, exercise, and diet of the United States, Italy, Holland, Greece, Japan, Finland, and Yugoslavia. Twenty years later, he published his findings in a landmark study called "The Seven Countries Study.

Keys' research found that the dietary choices of the people from the Mediterranean region allowed them to live a longer lifespan and one that kept them more physically active compared to other world populations. The people of Greece, in particular, ate a diet that consisted of healthy fats like seafood, nuts, olive oil, and fatty fish. Despite the amount of fat in these sources, their cardiovascular health stayed consistent without the risk factors for a heart attack or stroke. His study became a guideline for the United States to set its own nutritional standards, and he became known as the father of nutritional science.

With Keys' work leading the way, further research and clinical trials have been conducted on the Mediterranean diet which gives evidence for its health-improving properties. Not only will you lose weight, but you could lower your LDL "bad" cholesterol, lower your blood pressure, and decrease and stabilize blood sugar levels. With a decrease in these signs of cardiovascular heart disease, you can greatly reduce your risk of suffering from heart attack, stroke, or premature death.

It's important to point out that the Mediterranean diet cannot alone bring about these changes to someone's health. It will depend on a variety of other factors in their lifestyle such as genetics, physical exercise, smoking, obesity, drug use, *etc.* Part of the combination of the Mediterranean diet is incorporating physical exercise into your life. That's how it goes from the Mediterranean "diet" to a Mediterranean "lifestyle" that truly mimics the people of that region. The people of Greece tend to live an active lifestyle with some sort of daily physical activity they partake in. Whether that is walking, sailing, rowing, swimming, or hiking, coupling that physical exercise that with a healthy plant-based diet is what can bring about the beneficial health results. In our current environment, physical activity could mean a session at the gym or even just a walk around the block. It doesn't have to highly intensive, but the important part is incorporating some sort of physical activity in your day, so you can truly gain the benefits of following this diet.

Before we begin listing a rudimentary list of what you can and cannot eat, it's important to highlight that the Mediterranean region consists of many countries with their own unique dietary choices. With this diversity comes many varieties of recipes that you can incorporate into your dishes as long as you are still following the healthy tenets of the Mediterranean diet. This gives a basic outline of which foods you should include on your shopping list and then you can look for recipes from there! What does the basic Mediterranean diet look like?

- ➤ Your diet should consist heavily of whole grain bread, extra virgin olive oil, fresh fruits and vegetables, herbs and spices, nuts and seeds, fish and seafood
- ➤ You should moderately eat: poultry, cheese, egg, yogurt
- ➤ You should try to eat: red meat and organ meat rarely
- ➤ You should avoid the following: processed snacks, refined oils (canola oil or vegetable oil), refined grains (white bread), sugary drinks (juice, soda), processed meats (hot dogs, sausages, bacon), trans fats
- ➤ You should drink: water, wine

CHAPTER 2

THE BASIC PRINCIPLES AND THE FOODS TO PREFER

This leads to a variety of vegetables, fruit, whole grains, beans, healthy fats, red wine, beef, and fish. It's considered one of the healthiest diets.

FRUITS & VEGETABLES

The first part of the Mediterranean diet is fresh fruits and vegetables. Most vegetable sand fruits are low in fat and high in fiber, which make them heart healthy. They can help with weight loss too.

They're also full of antioxidants which can help to reduce inflammation and slow down the aging process.

The antioxidants include vitamins A, vitamin C, vitamin E and vitamin K. they can help to remove harmful free radicals that can cause the oxidation of LDL, also known as bad cholesterol.

WHOLE GRAINS

This is also a must for the Mediterranean diet. Refined grains have been stripped of nutrients during the refinement process, which means they aren't as healthy as whole grains which have more nutrition.

USING OLIVE OIL

Olive oil has a lot of monounsaturated fats which can protect against heart disease because it keeps LDL levels, bad cholesterol, low and HDL levels, good cholesterol, high. Most Mediterranean meals are prepared by liberally using olive oil. Also, on the Mediterranean diet most foods are grilled or baked, which is easier to do with olive oil.

FISH & CHICKEN

The Mediterranean diet often includes an abundance of fresh fish because of the proximity of the area to the sea. Fish has a lot of omega-3 fatty acids which have various heart healthy benefits including reducing triglycerides, inflammation and even cholesterol. There are various types of fish to choose from as well, including salmon, mackerel, herring, sardines, trout and albacore tuna. Chicken can also be used in pace of fish to replace red meat. It isn't as healthy as fish, but it does have lower saturated fats and cholesterol than red meat.

NUTS

Unsalted nuts are often eaten as a snack in Mediterranean countries. However, the US is more likely to go for things such as crackers or potato chips which have no health benefits. Nuts can also be included in desserts and savory dishes. Pine nuts can be used to make homemade pesto, and you'll find walnuts are often in bread dough. Nuts are a wonderful source of monounsaturated fat, and they're packed full of protein and fiber. They can also contain various minerals and vitamins which will help to improve your overall health.

RED WINE

Small amounts of alcohol is consumed with most meals, especially red wine, in Mediterranean countries. It's been proven that alcoholic drinks, such as red win, have healthy heart benefits. Red wine has an antioxidant called flavonoids which can prevent fatty deposits from building up in the artery walls. Even the American Heart Association recommends one to two drinks a day for men and women. These drinks are only supposed to be four ounces each.

SPICES

There are many spices and herbs that are used in the Mediterranean diet that also provide health benefits, including garlic. While these herbs and spices help to make the food taste great, their benefits to your health is the real magic.

The most common herbs and spices in this area are garlic, anise, basil, bay leaf, fennel, lavender, cumin, mint, marjoram, oregano, pepper, rosemary, sumaci, parsley, thyme and tarragon. Cutting down on salt can help to lower blood pressure, which is also a risk for heart disease, and these flavors help to lower your intake of salt? Garlic is a great way to spice up your meal, and you may not even know that the salt is missing!

DAIRY

Full fat dairy products, including cheese and whole milk, are eaten in small amounts in Mediterranean countries. This helps to keep the saturated fat intake down. However, traditional cheeses such as goat cheese and feta cheese are lower in fat than hard cheeses such as Cheddar, which is extremely popular in the US. There is also yogurt which is eaten more frequently by being included in various dishes and desserts which is very healthy. Eggs can also be eaten regularly, but egg yolk is limited in this diet. Egg yolk should be limited to four per week to help to control your saturated fat intake. Though, egg whites can be eaten much more often.

LEGUMES

The importance of legumes is also emphasized in the Mediterranean diet. These include beans, peas, lentils and snap peas. Legumes have a high fiber and protein count which is a great addition to your diet.

FOODS TO AVOID

You should reduce red meat in the Mediterranean diet since it can contribute to heart disease, but you don't have to avoid it completely. With this diet, you don't have to avoid anything completely, but there are certain items that should be reduced and eaten sparingly. When you want to eat something like red meat, try to choose a small portion of lean red meat instead, and keep it down to three to four times per month. Here are some more foods to limit or avoid all together if possible.

Added Sugars: This includes candies, ice cream, table sugar and soda.

Refined Grains: This includes pasta that's made of refined wheat and white bread.

Trans Fat: This can be found in various processed foods, but it's also in margarine!

Refined Oils: This includes cottonseed oil, vegetable oil, canola oil and soybean oil.

Processed Meats: Some common examples are processed hot dogs and sausages.

Highly Processed Foods: This includes anything that is labeled "diet", "low fat" or was obviously made in a factory. Remember that you should be concentrating on whole, natural ingredients.

Swapping Food Out

If you're trying to stick to a Mediterranean diet, you need to know what common food you're eating can be swapped with to help keep you on track.

Butter: Just swap it out for olive oil.

Salt: Just swap it out for a variety of herbs and spices instead.

Mayonnaise: Mayonnaise can be swapped out for mashed avocado.

Beer: It's better to switch to a glass or two of red wine which has heart benefits.

Beef: Beef isn't great for you, but you can usually swap it out for salmon which can easily be found at most grocery stores.

Potato Chips: Instead of munching on something that has no health benefits, choose a bag of mixed nuts. Just make sure they're unsalted.

Jam or Jelly: Swap it out for fresh fruit instead. You may want even to puree it in a food processor.

Rice or Bread: While you can eat whole wheat bread and some rice on the Mediterranean diet, cut it back. If you're trying to cut back try to switch for legumes instead.

Cakes & Cookies: Try vegetables and hummus for a healthy alternative that will curb your appetite.

THE TAKE AWAY

Now that you know what you should and shouldn't eat, you need to make sure that you avoid as much temptation as possible. Clean out your home from things that are too unhealthy, especially at the beginning of your dietary change. It can be hard to stick to a lifestyle change. You'll also need to keep in mind your portion control, and you'll need to start making some time for physical activity even if it's just twenty minutes a day.

TOP TIPS

You already know that starting a new diet can be hard, and the Mediterranean diet is no different. Here are some top tips so that you can be successful with your dietary change.

WHEN DINING OUT

You aren't going to be able to stop going out to eat just because you're on a diet, especially when it's going to be a lifestyle change. Of course, you should try to limit dining out whenever possible for the first month of your lifestyle change. However, when you do go out to eat, start by dividing your meal in half. Don't wait either. You'll want to divide your plate the moment it comes to you. Save half for later, so ask for a takeout container if at all possible. It's unlikely that you'll have food that fits your diet when eating out, so limiting your portion control is the first step in making sure you don't blow all of the hard work you've put in.

NEVER SKIP BREAKFAST

When dieting, skipping a meal can seem like a good idea but it isn't. Breakfast is one of the most commonly skipped meal because it's easier for you to wait for lunch than it is for someone to wait for dinner if they skip lunch. Though, skipping any meal can put your metabolism behind schedule. It's better to keep your refrigerator stocked with fruit and yogurt for small, light breakfasts that are also great on the go.

CHOP YOUR VEGETABLES

It's best to chop your vegetables in advance so that you can use them for snacks and quick lunches. Some of the best vegetables to keep on hand for this is bell peppers, celery, carrots and cucumbers. They're also perfect for dipping in hummus which is a healthy snack too!

SHOP LOCALLY

You may want to pay a visit to your local farmer's market as well. It's a great way to keep your house stocked full with seasonal vegetables that are sure to be fresh. It can also help to cut costs if you're shopping locally and seasonally. You shouldn't let your budget be your downfall when making an important lifestyle change, and shopping locally sourced food can help.

KEEP NUTS & SEEDS

It's just as important that you keep nuts and seeds on hand for a healthy alternative to chips, cookies and other processed foods. Some great choices are sunflower seeds, almonds or walnuts. Remember that these shouldn't be salted either!

USE FRUIT MORE

You can use fruit for dessert and even add some sweetness by drizzling honey or brown sugar over the top. Fresh fruit is a healthy snack when your stomach is hungry too, but the added, healthy sweetener should only be used when using it for dessert.

EAT SLOWER

You should savor your food if you want to make sure you aren't rushing through and eating more than you need to. If you cherish your time eating by sharing it with family and friends you will eat slower and consume less calories. You're also more likely to want to put in the extra effort to make a healthy, tasty meal which make take some time. That's why getting your family involved is also a healthful tip.

USE WHOLE GRAINS

You already know that whole grains are an essential part of the Mediterranean diet, so you need to switch to them for success. Minimally processed grains are healthier including couscous, bulgur, barley, oats rice, polenta, faro and millet.

MANAGE PORTIONS

The Mediterranean diet encourages portion control. Don't concentrate on counting calories. Instead, you need to concentrate on the quality of calories that you're eating. Calories are important, but your calorie type is much more important. This diet has nutrient dense food that will help you to stay full in the long run, so you don't have to eat a large amount of it. Always keep an eye on your plate size if you want to stay on track.

CHAPTER 3

SEASONAL SHOPPING: A KEY POINT.

A MEDITERRANEAN SHOPPING LIST

When you are shopping for food, you should make sure that you pick organic and fresh produce. Do not pick processed foods and avoid picking foods with high sugar and salt content.

What you add to your pantry depends on the kind of food you would like to prepare. However, here are a few essentials that will help you get started.

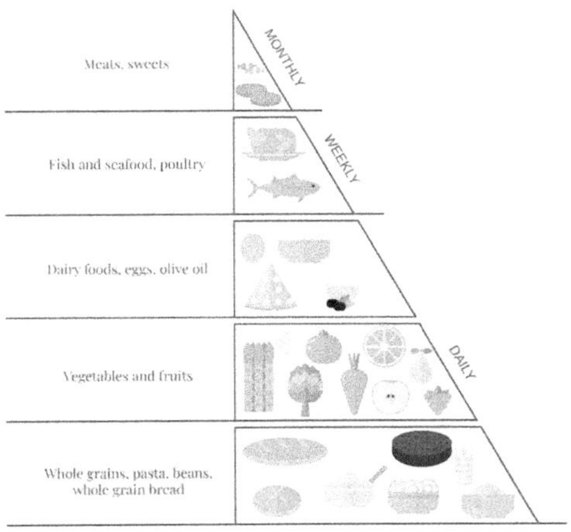

MEDITERRANEAN DIET

FRUITS

• apples • apricots • avocados • cherries • clementine's • dates • figs • grapefruits • grapes • melons • nectarines • olives • oranges • peaches • pears • pomegranates • strawberries • tangerines • tomatoes

VEGETABLES

• artichokes • arugula • beets • broccoli • Brussels sprouts • cabbage • carrots • celery • celeriac • chicory • collard greens • cucumbers • dandelion greens • eggplant • fennel • kale • leeks • lemons • lettuce • mache • mushrooms • mustard greens • nettles • okra • onions (red, sweet, white) • peas • peppers • potatoes • pumpkin • purslane • radishes • rutabaga • scallions • shallots • spinach • sweet potatoes • turnips • zucchini

NUTS, SEEDS, AND LEGUMES

• Almonds • cannellini beans • chickpeas • cashews • fava beans • green beans • hazelnuts • kidney beans • lentils • pine nuts • pistachios • sesame seeds • split peas • tahini sauce • walnuts

HERBS AND SPICES

• basil • bay leaf • black pepper • cloves • coriander • cumin • dill • fennel • garlic • lavender • marjoram • mint • oregano • parsley • paprika • rosemary • saffron • sage • savory • sumac • tarragon • thyme • turmeric

OTHER INCLUSIONS

• Frozen Vegetables: Choose only the healthy mixed veggie variety • Grains • All kinds of whole grains, including whole-grain bread and pasta • Fish: Salmon, tuna, sardines, herring, and sea bass • Shellfish varieties and shrimp • Free-range chicken • Baby potatoes and sweet potatoes • Cheese • Natural Greek yogurt • Olives • Pastured eggs • Goat, pork, and pastured beef • Extra virgin olive oil

A FEW TIPS TO REMEMBER

THE RULE OF THUMB

As a rule of thumb, make sure that you remove any unhealthy food that is not part of the Mediterranean diet or recommended by the list on this page. Make sure that you remove sweetened products, such as candy, baked goods, and soda. Get rid of refined grain products, artificially sweetened products, all processed foods, and crackers (especially those that have high salt content in them).

UPDATING THE LIST

The list above features some of the main ingredients used in Mediterranean diet and that should be included in your pantry. The list can get bigger depending on the region that influences you. For example, North African countries tend to use more cinnamon, cardamom, cloves, and nutmeg. If you find these ingredients in the recipes (or any other ingredients for that matter), then don't be alarmed; they are all part of the Mediterranean diet. If you feel that you might use some of the ingredients mentioned in the recipes more often, then you can include them in your pantry.

LEARN THE BASICS

Don't worry if you find yourself taking time to prepare the recipes. In many cases, the part that takes the most time is the preparations of the ingredients. Take your time and master the basics. The most important thing is that you are focused on having healthy food.

MEAL PLAN

You can even create your very own meal plan. It is quite simple really. Just combine various recipes from this book into a 14-day slot. Mix and match various breakfast, lunch, and dinner options until you have a plan that fits your preferences.

AND IT IS TIME TO LOOK AT SOME DELICIOUS RECIPES

If you are ready, then let's start looking at some lip-smacking recipes for your new Mediterranean diet.

MEDITERRANEAN DIET PYRAMID

Whole grains, vegetables, and fruits:

They're an integral part of the Mediterranean diet plan. The grains you should add to your diet should be non-refined whole grains such as quinoa and brown rice. Vegetables can include green leafy vegetables such as kale, spinach, broccoli, Brussels sprouts, cauliflower, and carrots.

Olive oil:

Olive oil is a very important part of the Mediterranean diet and is much healthier than other vegetable oils such as canola or sunflower oil. Use olive oil with every dish and replace butter and margarine with olive oil. Consume an average of ½ cup per week.

Beans, nuts, and seeds:

Beans, nuts, seeds, and lentils are a great source of protein. Use these ingredients as a substitute for red meat where possible. They provide a more filling, more affordable, and healthier source of protein compared to red meats.

Spices:

Use herbs and spices to flavor food instead of sodium-rich table salt. Get creative when flavoring food by combining fresh herbs with olive oil to marinade your food. Season dishes with fresh cracked black pepper for extra spiciness.

Fish and seafood:

The omega-3 oils found in fish is required for healthy brain development, and it helps reduce the risk of cardiovascular disease with regular consumption.

Poultry, eggs, cheese, and yogurt:

Include poultry, eggs, cheese, and yogurt in your daily diet. Always focus on moderate consumption of any dairy products and monitor their effects on you.

Meats:

Red meat should be kept to a minimum, as it isn't the healthiest diet option and can be substituted with legumes, bean, and seeds. When you do eat red meat, try to eat grass fed, organic red meat and keep it to a minimal amount of servings per week.

Red wine:

Many studies have shown that one glass of red wine per day can have multiple health benefits. The Mediterranean diet recommends enjoying one glass of red wine. Remember, more than two glasses can be detrimental to your health.

Physical activity and social interaction:

The Mediterranean lifestyle includes moderate amounts of daily physical activity and social interaction. Mediterranean's walk or cycle to work and lead very active lifestyles. Meals are also enjoyed as a family and are eaten over a longer period with plenty of conversation and laughs in between. If you can't walk or bike to work, try to take short walks when home and engage in as much physical activity -such as taking the stairs instead of the elevator-during your typical day as possible, Sit down at breakfast, lunch, and dinner and take time to savor your food. Try to taste every bite and identify the ingredients in each bite. Use dinnertime to talk to your family and discuss everyone's day, some goals for the week, your hobbies, and anything interesting you may have seen or heard that day.

CHAPTER 4

THE PRINCIPLES OF THE MEDITERRANEAN DIET

The principles of the Mediterranean diet are simple and easy to follow. You'll be pleased to discover that the Mediterranean diet is more about what you can and should eat than what you shouldn't eat.

EAT A PLANT-BASED DIET:

Build your meals around vegetables, fresh fruits, beans, and legumes. These whole foods are central to the health benefits of the Mediterranean diet. They provide energy in complex carbohydrates, antioxidants, vitamins, minerals, phytochemicals, and fiber. These nutrient-dense foods fill you up and keep you satisfied, thus controlling your weight while providing disease-fighting nutrients.

CHOOSE WHOLE GRAINS:

Avoid refined grains like white flour and rice. Choose whole grains such as whole wheat, brown rice, oats, barley, corn, quinoa, faro, bulgur, millet, and so on, including whole grain breads, and pasta. Whole grains are higher in nutrients, including minerals, vitamins, and fiber.

EAT FOODS THAT CONTAIN HEALTHY FATS, INCLUDING OLIVES, OLIVE OIL, NUTS, AND SEEDS:

Olive and olive oil are rich in heart-healthy monounsaturated fats and antioxidants. Add olives and olive oil to your pasta, salads, and stews, and have them as a snack. Nuts and seeds, such as almonds, cashews, pine nuts, hazelnuts, pistachios, pumpkin seeds, sesame seeds, and walnuts are also good sources of healthy fats. Avoid fats that are higher in saturated fats such as butter, cream, lard, or red meat. Completely avoid Tran's fats such as hydrogenated oils and margarine.

EAT FISH AND SEAFOOD:

Eat fish and seafood such as tuna, crab, squid, shrimp, sea bass, sardines, salmon, octopus, mussels, herring, cod, clams, bream, and anchovies.

LIMIT DAIRY, CHEESE, AND YOGURT.

MODERATION IS THE KEY:

It's vital to keep portion sizes in check when consuming high calorie and high saturated fat foods like cheese, red meat, refined grains, and foods sweetened with refined sugar.

TAKE TIME TO ENJOY LIFE AND BE PHYSICALLY ACTIVE:

The Mediterranean way of life is more relaxed than the typical American lifestyle. People in this coastal region take the time to enjoy meals with their families. They walk or bike to work instead of driving, and they take far more vacation time -all of which can reduce stress and contribute to good health.

CHAPTER 5

CEREALS AND GRAINS

On the Mediterranean diet, whole grains are high. However, if you are used to eating "white" starches, such as pasta, white rice, and white bread, then slowly shift to whole grains. You can begin with eating "light" whole-wheat bread, then slowly move to whole grain bread. If eating white rice, substitute any recipe that calls for it with brown rice. Replacing white rice with brown rice instantly increases your fiber consumption. You can also replace real potatoes with sweet potatoes and yams. Always choose whole-grain cereals.

HOW MUCH CAN I CONSUME ON THE MEDITERRANEAN DIET?

Men should at least 10.4 ounces and women at least 8.9 ounces of cereals and grains daily.

NUTS AND FRUITS

Nuts are perfect as snacks. They contain plenty of calories, but these calories come mainly from monounsaturated fat or MUFA, which are suitable fats that help the body lose weight. Studies show that if you eat 2 ounces of nuts instead of cookies, you will not gain any weight even though the nuts contain more calories than the cookies.

Fruits are the perfect sweet snacks. They satisfy your sweet tooth cravings without adding artificial sweeteners and additives into your diet. Pack your pantry and refrigerator with pears, apples, oranges, and more. Enjoying your fruits are juice is acceptable on the Mediterranean diet. Still, it's better to eat them since it will preserve their fiber content.

HOW MUCH CAN I CONSUME ON THE MEDITERRANEAN DIET?

Men should eat about 8.9 ounces daily while women should consume approximately 7.7 ounces a day.

LEGUMES

There are different kinds of vegetables that you can choose from to include in your diet. They are an excellent source of fiber and an excellent source of alternative protein. Legumes are also versatile. You can add them as an ingredient in your salads, soups, or main course recipes, or serve them as a side dish.

HOW MUCH CAN I CONSUME ON THE MEDITERRANEAN DIET?

Men should consume about 2.1 ounces, and women should eat approximately 1.75 ounces daily.

VEGETABLES

Veggies are the most important and the major component of the Mediterranean diet. There is no way you can eat too many vegetables.

You can eat a lot and still be within your recommended daily calorie intake. They help you feel full faster and longer.

One great way to increase your consumption of vegetables is to include them in your lunch and snack. Pile your favorite sandwich with onion, peppers, tomatoes, cucumbers, lettuce, and virtually anything you desire.

WHAT TO DO IF YOU DO NOT LIKE VEGGIES

Similar to fish, you can begin with the ones that you like. Think of all the veggies that you have already eaten and kept them on hand. Then slowly explore and add the ones that are less familiar to you.

HOW MUCH CAN I CONSUME ON THE MEDITERRANEAN DIET?

Men should eat at least 10.8 ounces and women at least 8.9 ounces a day.

THE MEDITERRANEAN DIET PYRAMID

The Mediterranean diet follows a food pyramid. Use the guide below to plan your dishes according to what you can eat daily or weekly.

DAILY MENU

Non-starchy vegetables (4-8 servings)

A serving size is:

- ➢ 1 cup raw vegetables
- ➢ One-half cup cooked vegetables

Non-starchy vegetables include all plants, except winter squash, peas, corn, and potatoes.

Whole grains and starchy vegetables (4-6 servings)

A serving size is:

- 1 slice bread, whole-wheat
- One-half cup corn, peas, potatoes, or winter squash
- 1/2 of a large-sized whole-grain bun
- 1 small-sized whole-grain roll
- 6 inches whole-wheat pita
- 6 whole-grain crackers
- One-half cup cooked whole-grain cereal
- One-half cup cooked barley, whole-wheat pasta, or brown rice

Fruits (2-4 servings)

A serving size is:

- One-half cup juice
- 1 small-sized fresh fruit
- One-fourth cup dried fruit

Always choose whole fruits, because they contain fiber and other nutrients. If you are using canned fruits, want the variety with no sugar or low sugar added. Consume no more than 8 ounces a day of fruit juices since even the unsweetened types are high in sugar.

Legumes and nuts (1-3 servings)

Aim for a 1-2 serving of nuts daily and 1-2 serving of vegetables daily.

A serving size is:

- ➢ 2 tablespoons sesame or sunflower seeds
- ➢ 1 tablespoon peanut butter
- ➢ 7 to 8 walnuts
- ➢ 20 peanuts
- ➢ 12 to 15 almonds
- ➢ One-fourth cup baked or refried beans, fat-free
- ➢ One-half cup kidney, lentils, navy beans, split peas, and pinto, soy, black, or garbanzo beans

WEEKLY MENU

Fish (2-3 servings)

A serving is 3 ounces or about the size of a deck of cards.

Dairy (1-3 servings)

A serving is:

- ➢ 1 cup of light yogurt, non-fat yogurt, or skim milk
- ➢ 10 ounces low-fat cheese

You can use soy cheese, soy milk, or soy yogurt instead.

Poultry (1-3 servings)

A serving is 3 ounces or about the size of a deck of cards. This is optional; you can opt not to add any poultry to your Mediterranean diet.

MONTHLY MENU

Eggs

You can eat as much as 4 egg yolks weekly. On the other hand, you can eat as much egg whites as you want.

Sweets

You can eat once a week or 3 to 4 times monthly.

Red meats (veal, lamb, and beef)

You can eat once a week or 3 to 4 times monthly.

Substitutions

If you want to replace a recipe ingredient with an ingredient that you like, then be sure to use an amount with the same or similar calorie count as the original. For example, you want to replace chicken with a salmon. A 2.6 ounces chicken has 176 calories, so you must replace it with 3 ounces of salmon, which contains 177 calories.

If you would like to substitute green beans with tomatoes, then replace 3/4 cup of green beans containing 26 calories with 1 cup cherry tomatoes containing 26 calories.

If you prefer strawberries instead of peaches, 2/3 cup peaches contain 44 calories, which you can replace with 1 cup strawberries containing 47 calories.

Important Reminders

The Mediterranean pyramid is a reliable guide for most adults. However, children, pregnant women, and people with special dietary needs may need nutritional supplements on a diet. In most circumstances, these special dietary needs can be accommodated on the Mediterranean diet.

THE PRECIOUS EXTRA VIRGIN OLIVE OIL.

This oil is a powerful and effective stimulant for weight loss. Its scent alone will help you feel fuller, making you eat less, and fewer calories. Olive oil is 75 percent monounsaturated fat or MUFA, the highest amount of any oil or food. Studies show that MUFA burns fat even if the person is not doing anything at all. Furthermore, studies show that consuming 1 spoonful of olive oil during breakfast increases fat oxidation and increases the body's ability to use fat as fuel or energy.

Furthermore, olive oil is condensed with oleic acid. This oil is a compound that helps halt hunger; which also makes you feel fuller for a longer time. Additionally, the oleic acid helps lower blood sugar level and control insulin.

THE FISH.

Fish

On the Mediterranean diet, you will eat more fish and less meat.

WHAT TO DO IF YOU DON'T LIKE FISH

Start with the kind you like or familiar with, then slowly try the kind you want less and less familiar with.

Fish are a better source of protein than meat. They also have lower fat content and seafood contains good fats, including omega-3 fatty acids, which are famous for reducing heart disease and stroke. Moreover, several studies indicate that consuming food rich in omega-3 fatty acids prevents certain types of cancer and helps alleviate problems with heart rhythm.

HOW MUCH CAN I CONSUME ON THE MEDITERRANEAN DIET?

Men should eat at least 1 ounce and women should eat at least 0.75 ounces daily. Please note, there have been concerns about mercury contamination lately. However, this does not mean that you can't consume seafood. You just need to be careful. The advantages of eating fish greatly outweigh the risk of contaminants. The Centers for Disease Control and Prevention recommends avoiding fish with more than 1.0 ppm (parts per billion) of mercury. Check the list of fish that you need to avoid. I have included a file on the subsequent pages of this book. It gives you.

LESS MEAT, MORE VEGETABLES.

Almost every person eats the same kinds of food every day. The key to a healthier body and weight loss is to consume more vegetables. Veggies are bulky with fewer calories. They are packed with micronutrients – antioxidants, phytochemicals, vitamins, and minerals that the body needs. Studies show that if a person's body is low in micronutrients, even just moderately little, its metabolism will slow down because it is not getting enough B vitamins, magnesium, and other nutrients. When the metabolism slows down, the body is not burning fat.

As you know, the human body is made up of around 60 to 70 percent water. When you are dehydrated, even just mildly dehydrated, the body will stop functioning correctly, including slowing down metabolism, digestion, and fat burning.

Eating veggies ensure you get the right amount of water because they are made up of 90 percent water. Furthermore, these green leafy vegetables are packed with fiber that fights off craving and hunger which aids you feel fuller longer.

ALTERNATIVE PROTEINS.

Swapping read meat with turkey, chicken, and fish lowers intake of saturated fat. You can also get your protein from beans, nuts, and other plants. Bream, herring, sardines, tuna, and salmon are good choices. Crustaceans and shellfish, including mussels, shrimps, and clams are also good sources.

Here's a quick way to reduce your meat consumption – make pasta and veggies the star of your meals and use meat as a flavoring or a condiment. Follow the recommended portion size for red meat. On the Mediterranean diet, shellfish and fish are rarely battered or fried.

CHAPTER 6

HOW TO SUCCEED ON THE MEDITERRANEAN DIET

Changing your diet can be quite a challenge, especially if you are adopting one that's very different from yours. Here are tips to make your transition to the Mediterranean Diet easier.

TASTE EVERY FLAVOR

More than a diet, the Mediterranean diet is a lifestyle that teaches you to enjoy and savor all the flavors of the food you eat. Avoid eating in front of the television since it will take your attention away from the food you are eating. Don't swallow everything in one bite. Instead, eat slowly, take your time, and taste every flavor. Eating slow will also tune your body with the food you eat. Enjoying your meals will even make you eat until you are just satisfied, and a prevent overeating.

KNOW YOUR IDEAL WEIGHT

Let the ideal weight for your height be your guide. Maintaining your weight gain is essential for good health. If you are overweight, then you need to exercise more and reduce the amount of food you eat and drink. Most people on a diet obsessively count calories, which can distract anyone from enjoying meals. Counting calories also do not work well in the long run.

BE WITH PEOPLE YOU LOVE

This Mediterranean diet is also based on the principles of enjoyment and pleasure. As much as possible, eat with friends and family. The happy company of others makes the food taste even better, and the laughter you share makes life even better.

CHOOSE A HEALTHY LIFESTYLE

Your overall health will not only depend on a healthy eating habit. Together with the Mediterranean diet, exercise and regular physical activities are also important. It doesn't have to be a workout in the gym. It could be as simple as taking the stairs instead of the elevator. Leisurely activities, such as walking, housework, or yard work are also good ways to move your body. You can even do running, aerobics, and other strenuous exercises.

MODERATION IS THE KEY

Unlike many diets that involve eliminating certain foods, the Mediterranean diet is a balanced diet that accommodates a wide range of drinks and food. The key is to eat moderately and wisely. On this diet, you can enjoy a small-sized slice of cake, a couple of slices of steak, and 1 to 2 glasses of wine.

FOLLOW THE RECOMMENDED FOOD FREQUENCY AND PORTION SIZE

This ensures that you get the right amount of food according to the ones that you can eat in large amounts and more frequently and the you need to eat in small quantities and less often.

HYDRATE

The body comprises 70 percent water, and proper hydration is essential to maintain energy levels, health, and well-being. Even mild dehydration will affect the processes in your body. The differences in metabolic rates, activity levels, and body type mean that some people need to drink more water than other people.

EAT EGGS

They are excellent sources of high-quality protein and are valuable for people who do not eat meat or vegetarian. Be sure to follow the recommended portions and frequency.

REDUCE SALT INTAKE

Use more herbs and spices and herbs to add flavor and aroma to food instead of salt. They add that distinct Mediterranean cuisine taste and are rich in antioxidants.

DRINK MODERATELY

Follow the recommended daily serving for each type of alcohol. Wine specifically had blood thinning effects, which makes the arteries less prone to clotting. They also contain antioxidants, which help prevent the build-up of low-density lipoprotein, or LDL in the arteries, in turn, avoiding the build-up of plaque in the arteries.

SNACK ON CHEESE, LOW-FAT DAIRY, SEEDS, AND NUTS

A handful of sunflower seeds, almonds, and walnuts make great meals. They are portable and on-the-go. Low-fat, calcium-rich cheese and fresh fruits are also great snacks on the go.

FRUITS FOR DESSERT

Most fruits are rich in antioxidants, fiber, and vitamin C. They are the healthiest desserts that will satisfy your sweet tooth. Discover and try out new fruits each week and widen your choices.

INCREASE WHOLE-GRAIN FOOD

It will take some time for your taste buds and stomach to adjust to whole-wheat and whole grain. Slowly replace your refined grain products with whole-grain ones. You can use whole-grain pasta blends or rice. You can also try mixing whole-grains with refined grained, half white and half whole-wheat. When your body has adjusted, then you can switch to whole-wheat and whole-grain completely.

PACK YOUR MEALS WITH VEGGIES

Most people do not consume enough veggies. Eat at least 3 to 4 servings a day. The more colorful, the better; more color means more vitamins and minerals. You can add them to your soups and omelets, enjoy them as a vegetable salad, or just roast them.

SWITCH PROTEINS

Swapping read meat with turkey, chicken, and fish lowers intake of saturated fat. You can also get your protein from beans, nuts, and other plants. Bream, herring, sardines, tuna, and salmon are good choices. Crustaceans and shellfish, including mussels, shrimps, and clams are also good sources.

Here's a quick way to reduce your meat consumption – make pasta and veggies the star of your meals and use meat as a flavoring or a condiment. Follow the recommended portion size for red meat. On the Mediterranean diet, shellfish and fish are rarely battered or fried.

USE PLANT OILS

Use them as your primary fat for cooking and baking. Eliminate all hydrogenated oils and oils containing trans-fat. As much as possible, replace butter and margarine with olive oil and other healthy oils, such as canola, soy, and peanut oil.

For a delicious yet healthy dipping for bread, season high-quality olive oil with balsamic vinegar. When cooking, do not let your oil get to smoking-hot because it will damage their nutritional properties and flavor. There are many interesting variations and many olive oil characteristics in the market, so experiment to find out which ones you can add to your diet.

A DAY ACCORDING TO THE MEDITERRANEAN DIET.

TO FILL UP ON ENERGY:

Breakfast

Green Eggs and Toast

TL;DR Mash an avocado with 1 tbsp minced mint, ½ tablespoon lemon juice, and a dash of pepper. Spread onto 2 pieces of whole-wheat toast and top with an egg. Sprinkle with 1 ½ ounces feta cheese and pepper.

Mid-morning Snack

Dates in a blanket

TL;DR Slice a piece of prosciutto into 4 lengthwise pieces. Wrap a fresh date in each piece of prosciutto. Sprinkle with pepper.

Lunch

Greek-Style Couscous

TL;DR Microwave 1 cup water and ¼ cup sundried tomatoes for 2 minutes. Let sit for 7 and drain water. Cook 210 grams couscous in 1 cup vegetable broth and 2 ½ tbsp water. Mix cooked couscous with 3 oz marinated artichoke hearts, 1 ½ cups cooked and diced chicken breast, ½ cup chopped parsley, sundried tomatoes, ¼ cup crumbled feta cheese, and a dash of pepper. Make 3 portions – saving 1 for Wednesday and Friday's lunch.

Afternoon Snack

10 almonds and 10 grapes (frozen grapes are awesome).

Dinner

Cheesy Eggplant Sandwich

TL;DR

Microwave ½ cup baby spinach until soft. Microwave sundried tomatoes, basil, and 1 ½ tbsp water until bubbling. Mix microwaved contents with ½ diced eggplant and ½ tbsp olive oil. Grill on medium-high until eggplant is slightly browned. Spread ½ tsp. olive oil over a piece of rustic Italian bread and grill. Top with grilled eggplant mixture, 2 tbsp. grated low-fat mozzarella, and ¾ tbsp. grated parmesan. Close grill lid over sandwich until cheese has melted.

Nutrient Breakdown

Calories – 1486
Fat in grams – 80
Carbs in grams – 198
Fiber in grams – 52
Protein in grams – 95

FOR THE HEART:

Breakfast

Good Morning Couscous

TL;DR Cook 1 ½ cups milk and an inch of a cinnamon stick over medium-high until bubbles form around edges. Take off heat and stir in ½ cup whole-grain couscous, 2 tbsp dried currants, and 2 tsp brown sugar. Cover and let sit for 15 minutes. Remove cinnamon stick and top with 1 tsp brown sugar. Eat half now and save half for Friday.

Mid-morning Snack

Baguette topped with Feta Cheese and Olives Marinade

TL;DR Mix together 1 1/3 cup black olives, ½ cup low-fat feta, 2 ½ tbsp olive oil, 2 cloves minced garlic, juice of 1 lemon, zest of 1 lemon, 1 tsp minced rosemary, a dash of cayenne pepper, and a dash of pepper.

Cover and refrigerate for a few hours before serving on 4 thin French baguette slices. Eat half today and save half for Friday's afternoon snack.

Lunch

One portion of the Greek-Style Couscous from Tuesday's lunch.

Afternoon Snack

½ cup plain low-fat Greek yoghurt topped with ½ cup blackberries and 1 tsp honey.

Dinner

Vegetarian Pasta Bolognese

TL;DR Fry 1 tbsp olive oil, ¼ cup diced carrot, 2 tbsp diced celery, and ½ small minced onion covered on medium heat. Once tender, add 2 cloves minced garlic, ½ bay leaf, and 2 tbsp white wine. Once wine evaporates, add ¼ cup mashed beans, tomatoes, and 1 tbsp parsley. Allow simmering until sauce is thick and then stir in 5 oz beans. Cook 4 ounces whole wheat pasta and drain. Combine pasta with sauce and sprinkle with ¼ cup grated parmesan cheese and 1 tbsp parsley. Eat ½ today, and save ½ for Friday's dinner.

Nutrient Breakdown

Calories – 1756
Fat in grams – 90
Carbs in grams – 220
Fiber in grams – 29
Protein in grams – 83

FOR SPORTS:

Breakfast

Fruity Yoghurt Parfait

TL;DR Bit by bit, scoop alternate layers of 6 oz low-fat yoghurt, 1 cup raspberries, and 2 tablespoons granola into a tall glass.

Mid-morning Snack

Ten baby carrots with ¼ cup Spicy Red Pepper Spread to dip.

Lunch

Classic Greek Salad

TL;DR Toss a salad of 1 head romaine, 1 red onion, 6 oz black olives, 2 sweet peppers, 2 large tomatoes, 1 cucumber, and 1 cup crumbled feta in a dressing of 6 tbsp olive oil, 1 tsp dried oregano, and a dash of pepper. Share half with a friend worthy of it!

Afternoon Snack

Sweet-Baked Banana

TL;DR Toss two ripe, sliced bananas in 4 tsp honey and ¾ tsp cinnamon. Bake on a lined baking sheet at 350F for 10-15 minutes. Split half with a friend worthy of it!

Dinner

Spanish Seafood Fried Rice

TL;DR Fry ¼ cup minced onion, ¼ cup diced sweet pepper, and 1 clove minced garlic in ½ tbsp olive oil over medium heat until tender. Add 1 cup instant brown rice, 2/3 cup vegetable broth, ¼ tsp thyme, a dash of saffron, and a dash of pepper. Once boiling, cover until vegetable broth evaporates. Add 8 oz shrimp, ½ cup peas, and arrange 8 oz mussels in a layer over top. Steam until mussels open. Remove from heat and let stand until vegetable broth is soaked up. Eat ½ today and save the rest for Saturday's dinner.

Nutrient Breakdown

Calories – 1301
Fat in grams – 46
Carbs in grams – 153
Fiber in grams – 25
Protein in grams – 54

CHAPTER 7

BREAKFAST RECIPES

1. EGG CASSEROLE WITH PAPRIKA

Preparation time: 10 minutes

Cooking time: 28 minutes

Servings: 4

INGREDIENTS

- 2 eggs, beaten
- 1 red bell pepper, chopped
- 1 chili pepper, chopped
- ½ red onion, diced
- 1 teaspoon canola oil
- ½ teaspoon salt
- 1 teaspoon paprika
- 1 tablespoon fresh cilantro, chopped
- 1 garlic clove, diced
- 1 teaspoon butter, softened
- ¼ teaspoon chili flakes

DIRECTIONS

1. Brush the casserole mold with canola oil and pour beaten eggs inside.
2. After this, toss the butter in the skillet and melt it over the medium heat.
3. Add chili pepper and red bell pepper.
4. After this, add red onion and cook the vegetables for 7-8 minutes over the medium heat. Stir them from time to time.
5. Transfer the vegetables in the casserole mold.
6. Add salt, paprika, cilantro, diced garlic, and chili flakes. Stir gently with the help of a spatula to get a homogenous mixture.
7. Bake the casserole for 20 minutes at 355F in the oven.
8. Then chill the meal well and cut into servings. Transfer the casserole in the serving plates with the help of the spatula.

NUTRITION:

Calories 68,
fat 4.5,
fiber 1,
carbs 4.4,
protein 3.4

2. CAULIFLOWER FRITTERS

Preparation time: 10 minutes

Cooking time: 10 minutes

Servings: 2

INGREDIENTS

- 1 cup cauliflower, shredded
- 1 egg, beaten
- 1 tablespoon wheat flour, whole grain
- 1 oz Parmesan, grated
- ½ teaspoon ground black pepper
- 1 tablespoon canola oil

DIRECTIONS

1. In the mixing bowl mix up together shredded cauliflower and egg.
2. Add wheat flour, grated Parmesan, and ground black pepper.
3. Stir the mixture with the help of the fork until it is homogenous and smooth.
4. Pour canola oil in the skillet and bring it to boil.
5. Make the cakes from the cauliflower mixture with the fingertips' help or use spoon and transfer in the hot oil.
6. Roast the fritters for 4 minutes from each side over the medium-low heat.

NUTRITION:

Calories 167,
fat 12.3,
fiber 1.5,

carbs 6.7,
protein 8.8

3. CREAMY OATMEAL WITH FIGS

Preparation time: 10 minutes

Cooking time: 20 minutes

Servings: 5

INGREDIENTS

- 2 cups oatmeal
- 1 ½ cup milk
- 1 tablespoon butter
- 3 figs, chopped
- 1 tablespoon honey

DIRECTIONS

1. Pour milk in the saucepan.
2. Add oatmeal and close the lid.
3. Cook the oatmeal for 15 minutes over the medium-low heat.
4. Then add chopped figs and honey.
5. Add butter and mix up the oatmeal well.
6. Cook it for 5 minutes more.
7. Close the lid and let the cooked breakfast rest for 10 minutes before serving.

NUTRITION:

Calories 222,
fat 6,
fiber 4.4,
carbs 36.5,
protein 7.1

4. BAKED OATMEAL WITH CINNAMON

Preparation time: 10 minutes

Cooking time: 25 minutes

Servings: 4

INGREDIENTS

- 1 cup oatmeal
- 1/3 cup milk
- 1 pear, chopped
- 1 teaspoon vanilla extract
- 1 tablespoon Splenda
- 1 teaspoon butter
- ½ teaspoon ground cinnamon
- 1 egg, beaten

DIRECTIONS

1. The big bowl mix up together oatmeal, milk, egg, vanilla extract, Splenda, and ground cinnamon.
2. Melt butter and add it in the oatmeal mixture.
3. Then add chopped pear and stir it well.
4. Transfer the oatmeal mixture in the casserole mold and flatten gently. Cover it with the foil and secure edges.
5. Bake the oatmeal for 25 minutes at 350F.

NUTRITION:

Calories 151,

fat 3.9,

fiber 3.3,

carbs 23.6,

protein 4.9

5. ALMOND CHIA PORRIDGE

Preparation time: 10 minutes

Cooking time: 30 minutes

Servings: 4

INGREDIENTS

- 3 cups organic almond milk
- 1/3 cup chia seeds, dried
- 1 teaspoon vanilla extract
- 1 tablespoon honey
- ¼ teaspoon ground cardamom

DIRECTIONS

1. Pour almond milk in the saucepan and bring it to boil.
2. Then chill the almond milk to the room temperature (or appx. For 10-15 minutes).
3. Add vanilla extract, honey, and ground cardamom. Stir well.
4. After this, add chia seeds and stir again.
5. Close the lid and let chia seeds soak the liquid for 20-25 minutes.
6. Transfer the cooked porridge into the serving ramekins.

NUTRITION:

Calories 150,
fat 7.3,
fiber 6.1,
carbs 18,
protein 3.7

6. COCOA OATMEAL

Preparation time: 10 minutes

Cooking time: 15 minutes

Servings: 2

INGREDIENTS

- 1 ½ cup oatmeal
- 1 tablespoon cocoa powder
- ½ cup heavy cream
- ¼ cup of water
- 1 teaspoon vanilla extract
- 1 tablespoon butter
- 2 tablespoons Splenda

DIRECTIONS

1. Mix up together oatmeal with cocoa powder and Splenda.
2. Transfer the mixture in the saucepan.
3. Add vanilla extract, water, and heavy cream. Stir it gently with the help of the spatula.
4. Close the lid and cook it for 10-15 minutes over the medium-low heat.
5. Remove the cooked cocoa oatmeal from the heat and add butter. Stir it well.

NUTRITION:

Calories 230,
fat 10.6,
fiber 3.5,

carbs 28.1,
protein 4.6

7. CINNAMON ROLL OATS

Preparation time: 7 minutes

Cooking time: 10 minutes

Servings: 4

INGREDIENTS

- ½ cup rolled oats
- 1 cup milk
- 1 teaspoon vanilla extract
- 1 teaspoon ground cinnamon
- 2 teaspoon honey
- 2 tablespoons Plain yogurt
- 1 teaspoon butter

DIRECTIONS

1. Pour milk in the saucepan and bring it to boil.
2. Add rolled oats and stir well.
3. Close the lid and simmer the oats for 5 minutes over the medium heat. The cooked oats will absorb all milk.
4. Then add butter and stir the oats well.
5. In the separated bowl, whisk together Plain yogurt with honey, cinnamon, and vanilla extract.
6. Transfer the cooked oats in the serving bowls.
7. Top the oats with the yogurt mixture in the shape of the wheel.

NUTRITION:

Calories 243, fat 20.2, fiber 1, carbs 2.8, protein 13.3

8. PUMPKIN OATMEAL WITH SPICES

Preparation time: 10 minutes

Cooking time: 13 minutes

Servings: 6

INGREDIENTS

- 2 cups oatmeal
- 1 cup of coconut milk
- 1 cup milk
- 1 teaspoon Pumpkin pie spices
- 2 tablespoons pumpkin puree
- 1 tablespoon Honey
- ½ teaspoon butter

DIRECTIONS

1. Pour coconut milk and milk in the saucepan. Add butter and bring the liquid to boil.
2. Add oatmeal, stir well with the help of a spoon and close the lid.
3. Simmer the oatmeal for 7 minutes over the medium heat.
4. Meanwhile, mix up together honey, pumpkin pie spices, and pumpkin puree.
5. When the oatmeal is cooked, add pumpkin puree mixture and stir well.
6. Transfer the cooked breakfast in the serving plates.

NUTRITION:

Calories 232,
fat 12.5,
fiber 3.8,

carbs 26.2,
protein 5.9

9. ZUCCHINI OATS

Preparation time: 10 minutes

Cooking time: 10 minutes

Servings: 4

INGREDIENTS

- 2 cups rolled oats
- 2 cups of water
- ½ teaspoon salt
- 1 tablespoon butter
- 1 zucchini, grated
- ¼ teaspoon ground ginger

DIRECTIONS

1. Pour water in the saucepan.
2. Add rolled oats, butter, and salt.
3. Stir gently and start to cook the oats for 4 minutes over the high heat.
4. When the mixture starts to boil, add ground ginger and grated zucchini. Stir well.
5. Cook the oats for 5 minutes more over the medium-low heat.

NUTRITION:

Calories 189,
fat 5.7,
fiber 4.7,
carbs 29.4,
protein 6

10. BREAKFAST SPANAKOPITA

Preparation time: 15 minutes

Cooking time: 1 hour

Servings: 6

INGREDIENTS

- 2 cups spinach
- 1 white onion, diced
- ½ cup fresh parsley
- 1 teaspoon minced garlic
- 3 oz Feta cheese, crumbled
- 1 teaspoon ground paprika
- 2 eggs, beaten
- 1/3 cup butter, melted
- 2 oz Phyllo dough

DIRECTIONS

1. Separate Phyllo dough into 2 parts.
2. Brush the casserole mold with butter well and place 1 part of Phyllo dough inside.
3. Brush its surface with butter too.
4. Put the spinach and fresh parsley in the blender. Blend it until smooth and transfer in the mixing bowl.
5. Add minced garlic, Feta cheese, ground paprika, eggs, and diced onion. Mix up well.
6. Place the spinach mixture in the casserole mold and flatten it well.

7. Cover the spinach mixture with remaining Phyllo dough and pour remaining butter over it.
8. Bake spanakopita for 1 hour at 350F.
9. Cut it into the servings.

NUTRITION:

Calories 190,
fat 15.4,
fiber 1.1,
carbs 8.4,
protein 5.4

CHAPTER 8

SALADS RECIPES

11. BULGUR SALAD

Preparation and Cooking Time 30 minutes

Servings 4

INGREDIENTS

- ➢ Vegetable stock - 2 cups
- ➢ Bulgur - 2 3 cup
- ➢ Garlic clove - 1, minced
- ➢ Cherry tomatoes - 1 cup, halved
- ➢ Almonds - 2 tbsp., sliced
- ➢ Dates - 1 4 cup, pitted and chopped
- ➢ Lemon juice - 1 tbsp.
- ➢ Baby spinach - 8 oz.
- ➢ Cucumber - 1, diced
- ➢ Balsamic vinegar - 1 tbsp.
- ➢ Salt and pepper - to taste
- ➢ Mixed seeds - 2 tbsp.

DIRECTIONS

1. Pour stock into sauce pan and heat until hot, then stir in bulgur and cook until bulgur has absorbed all stock.
2. Put in salad bowl and add remaining Ingredients:, stir well.
3. Add salt and pepper to suit your taste.
4. Serve and eat immediately.

12. TASTY TUNA SALAD

Servings 4

Preparation Time 15 minutes

INGREDIENTS

- Green olives - 1 4 cup, sliced
- Tuna in water - 1 can, drained
- Pine nuts - 2 tbsp.
- Artichoke hearts – 1 jar, drained and chopped
- Extra virgin olive oil - 2 tbsp.
- Lemon – 1, juiced
- Arugula - 2 leaves
- Dijon mustard - 1 tbsp.
- Salt and pepper - to taste

DIRECTIONS

1. Mix mustard, oil and lemon juice in a bowl to make a dressing. Combine the artichoke hearts, tuna, green olives, arugula and pine nuts in a salad bowl.
2. In a separate salad bowl, mix tuna, arugula, pine nuts, artichoke hearts and tuna.
3. Pour dressing mix onto salad and serve fresh.

13. SWEET AND SOUR SPINACH SALAD

Servings 4

Preparation Time 15 minutes

INGREDIENTS

- Red onions - 2, sliced
- Baby spinach leaves - 4
- Sesame oil - 1 2 tsp.
- Apple cider vinegar - 2 tbsp.
- Honey - 1 tsp.
- Sesame seeds - 2 tbsp.
- Salt and pepper - to taste

DIRECTIONS

1. Mix together honey, sesame oil, vinegar and sesame seeds in a small bowl to make a dressing. Add in salt and pepper to suit your taste.
2. Add red onions and spinach together in a salad bowl.
3. Pour dressing over the salad and serve while cool and fresh.

14. EASY EGGPLANT SALAD

Servings 4

Preparation Time 30 minutes

INGREDIENTS

- ➢ Salt and pepper - to taste
- ➢ Eggplant - 2, sliced
- ➢ Smoked paprika - 1 tsp.
- ➢ Extra virgin olive oil - 2 tbsp.
- ➢ Garlic cloves - 2, minced
- ➢ Mixed greens - 2 cups
- ➢ Sherry vinegar - 2 tbsp.

DIRECTIONS

1. Mix garlic, paprika and oil in a small bowl.
2. Place eggplant on a plate and sprinkle with salt and pepper to suit your taste. Next, brush oil mixture onto the eggplant.
3. Cook eggplant on a medium heated grill pan until brown on both sides. Once cooked, put eggplant into a salad bowl.
4. Top with greens and vinegar, serve and eat.

15. SWEETEST SWEET POTATO SALAD

Servings 4

Preparation and Cooking Time 30 minutes

INGREDIENTS

- Honey - 2 tbsp.
- Sumac spice - 1 tsp.
- Sweet potato - 2, finely sliced
- Extra virgin olive oil - 3 tbsp.
- Dried mint - 1 tsp.
- Balsamic vinegar – 1 tbsp.
- Salt and pepper - to taste
- Pomegranate - 1, seeded
- Mixed greens - 3 cups

DIRECTIONS

1. Place sweet potato slices on a plate and add sumac, mint, salt and pepper on both sides. Next, drizzle oil and honey over both sides.
2. Add oil to a grill pan and heat. Grill sweet potatoes on medium heat until brown on both sides.
3. Put sweet potatoes in a salad bowl and top with pomegranate and mixed greens.
4. Stir and eat right away.

16. DELICIOUS CHICKPEA SALAD

Servings 4

Preparation Time 15 minutes

INGREDIENTS

1. Chickpeas - 1 can, drained
2. Cherry tomatoes - 1 cup, quartered
3. Parsley - 1 2 cup, chopped
4. Red seedless grapes - 1 2 cup, halved
5. Feta cheese - 4 oz., cubed
6. Salt and pepper - to taste
7. Lemon juice - 1 tbsp.
8. Greek yogurt - 1 4 cup
9. Extra virgin olive oil - 2 tbsp.

DIRECTIONS

1. In a salad bowl, mix together parsley, chickpeas, grapes, feta cheese and tomatoes.
2. Add in remaining ingredients, seasoning with salt and pepper to suit your taste.
3. This fresh salad is best when served right away.

17. COUSCOUS ARUGULA SALAD

Servings 4

Preparation and Cooking Time 20 minutes

INGREDIENTS

- Couscous - 1 2 cup
- Vegetable stock - 1 cup
- Asparagus - 1 bunch, peeled
- Lemon - 1, juiced
- Dried tarragon - 1 tsp.
- Arugula - 2 cups
- Salt and pepper - to taste

DIRECTIONS

1. Heat vegetable stock in a pot until hot. Remove from heat and add in couscous. Cover until couscous has absorbed all the stock.
2. Pour in a bowl and fluff with a fork and then set aside to cool.
3. Peel asparagus with a vegetable peeler, making them into ribbons and put into a bowl with couscous.
4. Add remaining Ingredients and add salt and pepper to suit your taste.
5. Serve the salad immediately.

18. SPINACH AND GRILLED FETA SALAD

Servings 6

Preparation and Cooking Time 20 minutes

INGREDIENTS

- Feta cheese - 8 oz., sliced
- Black olives - 1 4 cup, sliced
- Green olives - 1 4 cup, sliced
- Baby spinach - 4 cups
- Garlic cloves - 2, minced
- Capers - 1 tsp., chopped
- Extra virgin olive oil - 2 tbsp.
- Red wine vinegar - 1 tbsp.

DIRECTIONS

1. Grill feta cheese slices over medium to high flame until brown on both sides.
2. In a salad bowl, mix green olives, black olives and spinach.
3. In a separate bowl, mix vinegar, capers and oil together to make a dressing.
4. Top salad with the dressing and cheese and it's is ready to serve.

19. CREAMY COOL SALAD

Servings 4

Preparation Time 15 minutes

INGREDIENTS

- Greek yogurt - 1 2 cup
- Dill - 2 tbsp., chopped
- Lemon juice - 1 tsp.
- Cucumbers - 4, diced
- Garlic cloves - 2, minced
- Salt and pepper - to taste

DIRECTIONS

1. Mix all Ingredients in a salad bowl.
2. Add salt and pepper to suit your taste and eat.

20. GRILLED SALMON SUMMER SALAD

Servings 4

Preparation and Cooking Time 30 minutes

INGREDIENTS

- Salmon fillets - 2
- Salt and pepper - to taste
- Vegetable stock - 2 cups
- Bulgur - 1 2 cup
- Cherry tomatoes - 1 cup, halved
- Sweet corn - 1 2 cup
- Lemon - 1, juiced
- Green olives - 1 2 cup, sliced
- Cucumber - 1, cubed
- Green onion - 1, chopped
- Red pepper - 1, chopped
- Red bell pepper - 1, cored and diced

DIRECTIONS

1. Heat a grill pan on medium and then place salmon on, seasoning with salt and pepper. Grill both sides of salmon until brown and set aside.
2. Heat stock in sauce pan until hot and then add in bulgur and cook until liquid is completely soaked into bulgur.
3. Mix salmon, bulgur and all other Ingredients in a salad bowl and again add salt and pepper, if desired, to suit your taste.
4. Serve salad as soon as completed.

CHAPTER 9

PASTA, RICE & GRAINS

21. DELICIOUS CHICKEN PASTA

Preparation Time: 10 minutes

Cooking Time: 17 minutes

Servings: 4

INGREDIENTS

- 3 chicken breasts, skinless, boneless, cut into pieces
- 9 oz whole-grain pasta
- 1/2 cup olives, sliced
- 1/2 cup sun-dried tomatoes
- 1 tbsp roasted red peppers, chopped
- 14 oz can tomatoes, diced
- 2 cups marinara sauce
- 1 cup chicken broth
- Pepper
- Salt

DIRECTIONS

1. Add all ingredients except whole-grain pasta into the instant pot and stir well.
2. Seal pot with lid and cook on high for 12 minutes.
3. Once done, allow to release pressure naturally. Remove lid.
4. Add pasta and stir well. Seal pot again and select manual and set timer for 5 minutes.
5. Once done, allow to release pressure naturally for 5 minutes then release remaining using quick release. Remove lid.
6. Stir well and serve.

NUTRITION:

Calories 615
Fat 15.4 g
Carbohydrates 71 g
Sugar 17.6 g
Protein 48 g
Cholesterol 100 mg

22. FLAVORS TACO RICE BOWL

Preparation Time: 10 minutes

Cooking Time: 14 minutes

Servings: 8

INGREDIENTS

- 1 lb ground beef
- 8 oz cheddar cheese, shredded
- 14 oz can red beans
- 2 oz taco seasoning
- 16 oz salsa
- 2 cups of water
- 2 cups brown rice
- Pepper
- Salt

DIRECTIONS

1. Set instant pot on sauté mode.
2. Add meat to the pot and sauté until brown.
3. Add water, beans, rice, taco seasoning, pepper, and salt and stir well.
4. Once done, release pressure using quick release. Remove lid.
5. Add cheddar cheese and stir until cheese is melted.
6. Serve and enjoy.

NUTRITION:

Calories 464
Fat 15.3 g
Carbohydrates 48.9 g
Sugar 2.8 g
Protein 32.2 g
Cholesterol 83 mg

23. FLAVORFUL MAC & CHEESE

Preparation Time: 10 minutes

Cooking Time: 10 minutes

Servings: 6

INGREDIENTS

- 16 oz whole-grain elbow pasta
- 4 cups of water
- 1 cup can tomatoes, diced
- 1 tsp garlic, chopped
- 2 tbsp olive oil
- 1/4 cup green onions, chopped
- 1/2 cup parmesan cheese, grated
- 1/2 cup mozzarella cheese, grated
- 1 cup cheddar cheese, grated
- 1/4 cup passata
- 1 cup unsweetened almond milk
- 1 cup marinated artichoke, diced
- 1/2 cup sun-dried tomatoes, sliced
- 1/2 cup olives, sliced
- 1 tsp salt

DIRECTIONS

1. Add pasta, water, tomatoes, garlic, oil, and salt into the instant pot and stir well.
2. Seal pot with lid and cook on high for 4 minutes.
3. Once done, allow to release pressure naturally for 5 minutes then release remaining using quick release. Remove lid.

4. Set pot on sauté mode. Add green onion, parmesan cheese, mozzarella cheese, cheddar cheese, passata, almond milk, artichoke, sun-dried tomatoes, and olive. Mix well.
5. Stir well and cook until cheese is melted.
6. Serve and enjoy.

NUTRITION:

Calories 519
Fat 17.1 g
Carbohydrates 66.5 g
Sugar 5.2 g
Protein 25 g
Cholesterol 26 mg

24. CUCUMBER OLIVE RICE

Preparation Time: 10 minutes

Cooking Time: 10 minutes

Servings: 8

INGREDIENTS

- 2 cups rice, rinsed
- 1/2 cup olives, pitted
- 1 cup cucumber, chopped
- 1 tbsp red wine vinegar
- 1 tsp lemon zest, grated
- 1 tbsp fresh lemon juice
- 2 tbsp olive oil
- 2 cups vegetable broth
- 1/2 tsp dried oregano
- 1 red bell pepper, chopped
- 1/2 cup onion, chopped
- 1 tbsp olive oil
- Pepper
- Salt

DIRECTIONS

1. Add oil into the inner pot of instant pot and set the pot on sauté mode.
2. Add onion and sauté for 3 minutes.
3. Add bell pepper and oregano and sauté for 1 minute.
4. Add rice and broth and stir well.
5. Seal pot with lid and cook on high for 6 minutes.

6. Once done, allow to release pressure naturally for 10 minutes then release remaining using quick release. Remove lid.
7. Add remaining ingredients and stir everything well to mix.
8. Serve immediately and enjoy it.

NUTRITION:

Calories 229
Fat 5.1 g
Carbohydrates 40.2 g
Sugar 1.6 g
Protein 4.9 g
Cholesterol 0 mg

25. FLAVORS HERB RISOTTO

Preparation Time: 10 minutes

Cooking Time: 15 minutes

Servings: 4

INGREDIENTS

- 2 cups of rice
- 2 tbsp parmesan cheese, grated
- 3.5 oz heavy cream
- 1 tbsp fresh oregano, chopped
- 1 tbsp fresh basil, chopped
- 1/2 tbsp sage, chopped
- 1 onion, chopped
- 2 tbsp olive oil
- 1 tsp garlic, minced
- 4 cups vegetable stock
- Pepper
- Salt

DIRECTIONS

1. Add oil into the inner pot of instant pot and set the pot on sauté mode.
2. Add garlic and onion and sauté for 2-3 minutes.
3. Add remaining ingredients except for parmesan cheese and heavy cream and stir well.
4. Seal pot with lid and cook on high for 12 minutes.

5. Once done, allow to release pressure naturally for 10 minutes then release remaining using quick release. Remove lid.
6. Stir in cream and cheese and serve.

NUTRITION:

Calories 514
Fat 17.6 g
Carbohydrates 79.4 g
Sugar 2.1 g
Protein 8.8 g
Cholesterol 36 mg

26. DELICIOUS PASTA PRIMAVERA

Preparation Time: 10 minutes

Cooking Time: 4 minutes

Servings: 4

INGREDIENTS

- 8 oz whole wheat penne pasta
- 1 tbsp fresh lemon juice
- 2 tbsp fresh parsley, chopped
- 1/4 cup almonds slivered
- 1/4 cup parmesan cheese, grated
- 14 oz can tomatoes, diced
- 1/2 cup prunes
- 1/2 cup zucchini, chopped
- 1/2 cup asparagus, cut into 1-inch pieces
- 1/2 cup carrots, chopped
- 1/2 cup broccoli, chopped
- 1 3/4 cups vegetable stock
- Pepper
- Salt

DIRECTIONS

1. Add stock, pars, tomatoes, prunes, zucchini, asparagus, carrots, and broccoli into the instant pot and stir well.
2. Seal pot with lid and cook on high for 4 minutes.
3. Once done, release pressure using quick release. Remove lid.
4. Add remaining ingredients and stir well and serve.

NUTRITION:

Calories 303

Fat 2.6 g

Carbohydrates 63.5 g

Sugar 13.4 g

Protein 12.8 g

Cholesterol 1 mg

27. ROASTED PEPPER PASTA

Preparation Time: 10 minutes

Cooking Time: 13 minutes

Servings: 6

INGREDIENTS

- 1 lb whole wheat penne pasta
- 1 tbsp Italian seasoning
- 4 cups vegetable broth
- 1 tbsp garlic, minced
- 1/2 onion, chopped
- 14 oz jar roasted red peppers
- 1 cup feta cheese, crumbled
- 1 tbsp olive oil
- Pepper
- Salt

DIRECTIONS

1. Add roasted pepper into the blender and blend until smooth.
2. Add oil into the inner pot of instant pot and set the pot on sauté mode.
3. Add garlic and onion and sauté for 2-3 minutes.
4. Add blended roasted pepper and sauté for 2 minutes.
5. Add remaining ingredients except feta cheese and stir well.
6. Seal pot with lid and cook on high for 8 minutes.

7. Once done, allow to release pressure naturally for 5 minutes then release remaining using quick release. Remove lid.
8. Top with feta cheese and serve.

NUTRITION:

Calories 459
Fat 10.6 g
Carbohydrates 68.1 g
Sugar 2.1 g
Protein 21.3 g
Cholesterol 24 mg

28. CHEESE BASIL TOMATO RICE

Preparation Time: 10 minutes

Cooking Time: 26 minutes

Servings: 8

INGREDIENTS

- 1 1/2 cups brown rice
- 1 cup parmesan cheese, grated
- 1/4 cup fresh basil, chopped
- 2 cups grape tomatoes, halved
- 8 oz can tomato sauce
- 1 3/4 cup vegetable broth
- 1 tbsp garlic, minced
- 1/2 cup onion, diced
- 1 tbsp olive oil
- Pepper
- Salt

DIRECTIONS

1. Add oil into the inner pot of instant pot and set the pot on sauté mode.
2. Add garlic and onion and sauté for 4 minutes.
3. Add rice, tomato sauce, broth, pepper, and salt and stir well.
4. Seal pot with lid and cook on high for 22 minutes.
5. Once done, allow to release pressure naturally for 10 minutes then release remaining using quick release. Remove lid.

6. Add remaining ingredients and stir well.
7. Serve and enjoy.

NUTRITION:

Calories 208
Fat 5.6 g
Carbohydrates 32.1 g
Sugar 2.8 g
Protein 8.3 g
Cholesterol 8 mg

29. MAC & CHEESE

Preparation Time: 10 minutes

Cooking Time: 4 minutes

Servings: 8

INGREDIENTS

- 1 lb whole grain pasta
- 1/2 cup parmesan cheese, grated
- 4 cups cheddar cheese, shredded
- 1 cup milk
- 1/4 tsp garlic powder
- 1/2 tsp ground mustard
- 2 tbsp olive oil
- 4 cups of water
- Pepper
- Salt

DIRECTIONS

1. Add pasta, garlic powder, mustard, oil, water, pepper, and salt into the instant pot.
2. Seal pot with lid and cook on high for 4 minutes.
3. Once done, release pressure using quick release. Remove lid.
4. Add remaining ingredients and stir well and serve.

NUTRITION:

Calories 509

Fat 25.7 g

Carbohydrates 43.8 g

Sugar 3.8 g

Protein 27.3 g

Cholesterol 66 mg

30. TUNA PASTA

Preparation Time: 10 minutes

Cooking Time: 8 minutes

Servings: 6

INGREDIENTS

- 10 oz can tuna, drained
- 15 oz whole wheat rotini pasta
- 4 oz mozzarella cheese, cubed
- 1/2 cup parmesan cheese, grated
- 1 tsp dried basil
- 14 oz can tomatoes, diced
- 4 cups vegetable broth
- 1 tbsp garlic, minced
- 8 oz mushrooms, sliced
- 2 zucchini, sliced
- 1 onion, chopped
- 2 tbsp olive oil
- Pepper
- Salt

DIRECTIONS

1. Add oil into the inner pot of instant pot and set the pot on sauté mode.
2. Add mushrooms, zucchini, and onion and sauté until onion is softened.
3. Add garlic and sauté for a minute.
4. Add pasta, basil, tuna, tomatoes, and broth and stir well.

5.   Seal pot with lid and cook on high for 4 minutes.

6.   Once done, allow to release pressure naturally for 5 minutes then release remaining using quick release. Remove lid.

7.   Add remaining ingredients and stir well and serve.

NUTRITION:

Calories 346
Fat 11.9 g
Carbohydrates 31.3 g
Sugar 6.3 g
Protein 6.3 g
Cholesterol 30 mg

CHAPTER 10

SEAFOOD & FISH RECIPES

31. MEDITERRANEAN FISH FILLETS

Preparation Time: 10 minutes

Cooking Time: 3 minutes

Servings: 4

INGREDIENTS

- 4 cod fillets
- 1 lb grape tomatoes, halved
- 1 cup olives, pitted and sliced
- 2 tbsp capers
- 1 tsp dried thyme
- 2 tbsp olive oil
- 1 tsp garlic, minced
- Pepper
- Salt

DIRECTIONS

1. Pour 1 cup water into the instant pot then place steamer rack in the pot.
2. Spray heat-safe baking dish with cooking spray.
3. Add half grape tomatoes into the dish and season with pepper and salt.
4. Arrange fish fillets on top of cherry tomatoes. Drizzle with oil and season with garlic, thyme, capers, pepper, and salt.
5. Spread olives and remaining grape tomatoes on top of fish fillets.
6. Place dish on top of steamer rack in the pot.
7. Seal pot with a lid and select manual and cook on high for 3 minutes.
8. Once done, release pressure using quick release. Remove lid.
9. Serve and enjoy.

NUTRITION:

Calories 212
Fat 11.9 g
Carbohydrates 7.1 g
Sugar 3 g
Protein 21.4 g
Cholesterol 55 mg

32. FLAVORS CIOPPINO

Preparation Time: 10 minutes

Cooking Time: 5 minutes

Servings: 6

INGREDIENTS

- 1 lb codfish, cut into chunks
- 1 1/2 lbs shrimp
- 28 oz can tomatoes, diced
- 1 cup dry white wine
- 1 bay leaf
- 1 tsp cayenne
- 1 tsp oregano
- 1 shallot, chopped
- 1 tsp garlic, minced
- 1 tbsp olive oil
- 1/2 tsp salt

DIRECTIONS

1. Add oil into the inner pot of instant pot and set the pot on sauté mode.
2. Add shallot and garlic and sauté for 2 minutes.
3. Add wine, bay leaf, cayenne, oregano, and salt and cook for 3 minutes.
4. Add remaining ingredients and stir well.
5. Seal pot with a lid and select manual and cook on low for 0 minutes.

6. Once done, release pressure using quick release. Remove lid.
7. Serve and enjoy.

NUTRITION:

Calories 281

Fat 5 g
Carbohydrates 10.5 g
Sugar 4.9 g
Protein 40.7 g
Cholesterol 266 mg

33. DELICIOUS SHRIMP ALFREDO

Preparation Time: 10 minutes

Cooking Time: 3 minutes

Servings: 4

INGREDIENTS

- 12 shrimp, remove shells
- 1 tbsp garlic, minced
- 1/4 cup parmesan cheese
- 2 cups whole wheat rotini noodles
- 1 cup fish broth
- 15 oz alfredo sauce
- 1 onion, chopped
- Salt

DIRECTIONS

1. Add all ingredients except parmesan cheese into the instant pot and stir well.
2. Seal pot with lid and cook on high for 3 minutes.
3. Once done, release pressure using quick release. Remove lid.
4. Stir in cheese and serve.

NUTRITION:

Calories 669

Fat 23.1 g

Carbohydrates 76 g

Sugar 2.4 g

Protein 37.8 g

Cholesterol 190 mg

34. TOMATO OLIVE FISH FILLETS

Preparation Time: 10 minutes

Cooking Time: 8 minutes

Servings: 4

INGREDIENTS

- 2 lbs halibut fish fillets
- 2 oregano sprigs
- 2 rosemary sprigs
- 2 tbsp fresh lime juice
- 1 cup olives, pitted
- 28 oz can tomatoes, diced
- 1 tbsp garlic, minced
- 1 onion, chopped
- 2 tbsp olive oil

DIRECTIONS

1. Add oil into the inner pot of instant pot and set the pot on sauté mode.
2. Add onion and sauté for 3 minutes.
3. Add garlic and sauté for a minute.
4. Add lime juice, olives, herb sprigs, and tomatoes and stir well.
5. Seal pot with lid and cook on high for 3 minutes.
6. Once done, release pressure using quick release. Remove lid.
7. Add fish fillets and seal pot again with lid and cook on high for 2 minutes.

8. Once done, release pressure using quick release. Remove lid.
9. Serve and enjoy.

NUTRITION:

Calories 333
Fat 19.1 g
Carbohydrates 31.8 g
Sugar 8.4 g
Protein 13.4 g
Cholesterol 5 mg

35. SHRIMP SCAMPI

Preparation Time: 10 minutes

Cooking Time: 8 minutes

Servings: 6

INGREDIENTS

- 1 lb whole wheat penne pasta
- 1 lb frozen shrimp
- 2 tbsp garlic, minced
- 1/4 tsp cayenne
- 1/2 tbsp Italian seasoning
- 1/4 cup olive oil
- 3 1/2 cups fish stock
- Pepper
- Salt

DIRECTIONS

1. Add all ingredients into the inner pot of instant pot and stir well.
2. Seal pot with lid and cook on high for 6 minutes.
3. Once done, release pressure using quick release. Remove lid.
4. Stir well and serve.

NUTRITION:

Calories 435

Fat 12.6 g

Carbohydrates 54.9 g

Sugar 0.1 g

Protein 30.6 g

Cholesterol 116 mg

36. EASY SALMON STEW

Preparation Time: 10 minutes

Cooking Time: 8 minutes

Servings: 6

INGREDIENTS

- 2 lbs salmon fillet, cubed
- 1 onion, chopped
- 2 cups fish broth
- 1 tbsp olive oil
- Pepper
- salt

DIRECTIONS

1. Add oil into the inner pot of instant pot and set the pot on sauté mode.
2. Add onion and sauté for 2 minutes.
3. Add remaining ingredients and stir well.
4. Seal pot with lid and cook on high for 6 minutes.
5. Once done, release pressure using quick release. Remove lid.
6. Stir and serve.

NUTRITION:

Calories 243

Fat 12.6 g

Carbohydrates 0.8 g

Sugar 0.3 g

Protein 31 g

Cholesterol 78 mg

37. ITALIAN TUNA PASTA

Preparation Time: 10 minutes

Cooking Time: 5 minutes

Servings: 6

INGREDIENTS

- 15 oz whole wheat pasta
- 2 tbsp capers
- 3 oz tuna
- 2 cups can tomatoes, crushed
- 2 anchovies
- 1 tsp garlic, minced
- 1 tbsp olive oil
- Salt

DIRECTIONS

1. Add oil into the inner pot of instant pot and set the pot on sauté mode.
2. Add anchovies and garlic and sauté for 1 minute.
3. Add remaining ingredients and stir well. Pour enough water into the pot to cover the pasta.
4. Seal pot with a lid and select manual and cook on low for 4 minutes.
5. Once done, release pressure using quick release. Remove lid.
6. Stir and serve.

NUTRITION:

Calories 339

Fat 6 g

Carbohydrates 56.5 g

Sugar 5.2 g

Protein 15.2 g

Cholesterol 10 mg

38. GARLICKY CLAMS

Preparation Time: 10 minutes

Cooking Time: 5 minutes

Servings: 4

INGREDIENTS

- 3 lbs clams, clean
- 4 garlic cloves
- 1/4 cup olive oil
- 1/2 cup fresh lemon juice
- 1 cup white wine
- Pepper
- Salt

DIRECTIONS

1. Add oil into the inner pot of instant pot and set the pot on sauté mode.
2. Add garlic and sauté for 1 minute.
3. Add wine and cook for 2 minutes.
4. Add remaining ingredients and stir well.
5. Seal pot with lid and cook on high for 2 minutes.
6. Once done, allow to release pressure naturally. Remove lid.
7. Serve and enjoy.

NUTRITION:

Calories 332

Fat 13.5 g

Carbohydrates 40.5 g

Sugar 12.4 g

Protein 2.5 g

Cholesterol 0 mg

39. DELICIOUS FISH TACOS

Preparation Time: 10 minutes

Cooking Time: 8 minutes

Servings: 8

INGREDIENTS

- 4 tilapia fillets
- 1/4 cup fresh cilantro, chopped
- 1/4 cup fresh lime juice
- 2 tbsp paprika
- 1 tbsp olive oil
- Pepper
- Salt

DIRECTIONS

1. Pour 2 cups of water into the instant pot then place steamer rack in the pot.
2. Place fish fillets on parchment paper.
3. Season fish fillets with paprika, pepper, and salt and drizzle with oil and lime juice.
4. Fold parchment paper around the fish fillets and place them on a steamer rack in the pot.
5. Seal pot with lid and cook on high for 8 minutes.
6. Once done, release pressure using quick release. Remove lid.
7. Remove fish packet from pot and open it.
8. Shred the fish with a fork and serve.

NUTRITION:

Calories 67

Fat 2.5 g

Carbohydrates 1.1 g

Sugar 0.2 g

Protein 10.8 g

Cholesterol 28 mg

40. PESTO FISH FILLET

Preparation Time: 10 minutes

Cooking Time: 8 minutes

Servings: 4

INGREDIENTS

- 4 halibut fillets
- 1/2 cup water
- 1 tbsp lemon zest, grated
- 1 tbsp capers
- 1/2 cup basil, chopped
- 1 tbsp garlic, chopped
- 1 avocado, peeled and chopped
- Pepper
- Salt

DIRECTIONS

1. Add lemon zest, capers, basil, garlic, avocado, pepper, and salt into the blender blend until smooth.
2. Place fish fillets on aluminum foil and spread a blended mixture on fish fillets.
3. Fold foil around the fish fillets.
4. Pour water into the instant pot and place trivet in the pot.
5. Place foil fish packet on the trivet.
6. Seal pot with lid and cook on high for 8 minutes.
7. Once done, allow to release pressure naturally. Remove lid.
8. Serve and enjoy.

NUTRITION:

Calories 426

Fat 16.6 g

Carbohydrates 5.5 g

Sugar 0.4 g

Protein 61.8 g

Cholesterol 93 mg

CHAPTER 11

VEGETABLES

41. GARLIC BASIL ZUCCHINI

Preparation Time: 10 minutes

Cooking Time: 8 minutes

Servings: 4

INGREDIENTS

- 14 oz zucchini, sliced
- 1/4 cup fresh basil, chopped
- 1/2 tsp red pepper flakes
- 14 oz can tomatoes, chopped
- 1 tsp garlic, minced
- 1/2 onion, chopped
- 1/4 cup feta cheese, crumbled
- 1 tbsp olive oil
- Salt

DIRECTIONS

1. Add onion and garlic and sauté for 2 minutes.
2. Add remaining ingredients except feta cheese and stir well.
3. Seal pot with lid and cook on high for 6 minutes.
4. Once done, allow to release pressure naturally. Remove lid.
5. Top with feta cheese and serve.

NUTRITION:

Calories 99
Fat 5.7 g
Carbohydrates 10.4 g
Sugar 6.1 g
Protein 3.7 g
Cholesterol 8 mg

42. FETA GREEN BEANS

Preparation Time: 10 minutes

Cooking Time: 15 minutes

Servings: 4

INGREDIENTS

- 1 1/2 lbs green beans, trimmed
- 1/4 cup feta cheese, crumbled
- 28 oz can tomatoes, crushed
- 2 tsp oregano
- 1 tsp cumin
- 1/2 cup water
- 1 tbsp olive oil
- 1 tbsp garlic, minced
- 1 onion, chopped
- 1 lb baby potatoes, clean and cut into chunks
- Pepper
- Salt

DIRECTIONS

1. Add onion and garlic and sauté for 3-5 minutes.
2. Add remaining ingredients except feta cheese and stir well.
3. Seal pot with lid and cook on high for 10 minutes.
4. Once done, allow to release pressure naturally for 5 minutes then release remaining using quick release. Remove lid.
5. Top with feta cheese and serve.

NUTRITION:

Calories 234

Fat 6.1 g

Carbohydrates 40.7 g

Sugar 10.7 g

Protein 9.7 g

Cholesterol 8 mg

43. GARLIC PARMESAN ARTICHOKES

Preparation Time: 12 minutes

Cooking Time: 10 minutes

Servings: 4

INGREDIENTS

- 4 artichokes, wash, trim, and cut top
- 1/2 cup vegetable broth
- 1/4 cup parmesan cheese, grated
- 1 tbsp olive oil
- 2 tsp garlic, minced

DIRECTIONS

1. Pour broth into the instant pot then place steamer rack in the pot.
2. Place artichoke steam side down on steamer rack into the pot.
3. Sprinkle garlic and grated cheese on top of artichokes and season with salt. Drizzle oil over artichokes.
4. Seal pot with lid and cook on high for 10 minutes.
5. Once done, release pressure using quick release. Remove lid.
6. Serve and enjoy.

NUTRITION:

Calories 132

Fat 5.2 g

Carbohydrates 17.8 g

Sugar 1.7 g

Protein 7.9 g

Cholesterol 4 mg

44. DELICIOUS PEPPER ZUCCHINI

Preparation Time: 10 minutes

Cooking Time: 10 minutes

Servings: 6

INGREDIENTS

- 1 zucchini, sliced
- 2 poblano peppers, sliced
- 1 tbsp sour cream
- 1/2 tsp ground cumin
- 1 yellow squash, sliced
- 1 tbsp garlic, minced
- 1/2 onion, sliced
- 1 tbsp olive oil
- Salt

DIRECTIONS

1. Add poblano peppers and sauté for 5 minutes
2. Add onion and garlic and sauté for 3 minutes.
3. Add remaining ingredients except for sour cream and stir well.
4. Seal pot with lid and cook on high for 2 minutes.
5. Once done, release pressure using quick release. Remove lid.
6. Add sour cream and stir well and serve.

NUTRITION:

Calories 42

Fat 2.9 g

Carbohydrates 4 g

Sugar 1.7 g

Protein 1 g

Cholesterol 1 mg

45. CELERY CARROT BROWN LENTILS

Preparation Time: 10 minutes

Cooking Time: 25 minutes

Servings: 6

INGREDIENTS

- 2 cups dry brown lentils, rinsed and drained
- 2 1/2 cups vegetable stock
- 2 tomatoes, chopped
- 1/2 tsp red pepper flakes
- 1/2 tsp ground cinnamon
- 1 bay leaf
- 1 tbsp tomato paste
- 2 celery stalks, diced
- 2 carrots, grated
- 1 tbsp garlic, minced
- 2 onions, chopped
- 1/4 cup olive oil
- Pepper
- Salt

DIRECTIONS

1. Add celery, carrot, garlic, onion, pepper, and salt and sauté for 3 minutes.
2. Add remaining ingredients and stir everything well.
3. Seal pot with lid and cook on high for 22 minutes.
4. Once done, release pressure using quick release. Remove lid.
5. Stir well and serve.

NUTRITION:

Calories 137

Fat 8.8 g

Carbohydrates 12.3 g

Sugar 4.7 g

Protein 3.1 g

Cholesterol 0 mg

46. LEMON ARTICHOKES

Preparation Time: 10 minutes

Cooking Time: 20 minutes

Servings: 4

INGREDIENTS

- 4 artichokes, trim and cut the top
- 1/4 cup fresh lemon juice
- 2 cups vegetable stock
- 1 tsp lemon zest, grated
- Pepper
- Salt

DIRECTIONS

1. Pour the stock into the instant pot then place steamer rack in the pot.
2. Place artichoke steam side down on steamer rack into the pot.
3. Sprinkle lemon zest over artichokes. Season with pepper and salt.
4. Pour lemon juice over artichokes.
5. Seal pot with lid and cook on high for 20 minutes.
6. Once done, allow to release pressure naturally for 5 minutes then release remaining using quick release. Remove lid.
7. Serve and enjoy.

NUTRITION:

Calories 83

Fat 0.4 g

Carbohydrates 17.9 g

Sugar 2.3 g

Protein 5.6 g

Cholesterol 0 mg

47. EASY CHILI PEPPER ZUCCHINIS

Preparation Time: 10 minutes

Cooking Time: 10 minutes

Servings: 4

INGREDIENTS

- 4 zucchinis, cut into cubes
- 1/2 tsp red pepper flakes
- 1/2 tsp cayenne
- 1 tbsp chili powder
- 1/4 cup vegetable stock
- Salt

DIRECTIONS

1. Seal pot with lid and cook on high for 10 minutes.
2. Once done, allow to release pressure naturally for 10 minutes then release remaining using quick release. Remove lid.
3. Stir and serve.

NUTRITION:

Calories 38
Fat 0.7 g
Carbohydrates 8.8 g
Sugar 3.6 g
Protein 2.7 g
Cholesterol 0 mg

48. DELICIOUS OKRA

Preparation Time: 10 minutes

Cooking Time: 10 minutes

Servings: 4

INGREDIENTS

- 2 cups okra, chopped
- 2 tbsp fresh dill, chopped
- 1 tbsp paprika
- 1 cup can tomato, crushed
- Pepper
- Salt

DIRECTIONS

1. Seal pot with lid and cook on high for 10 minutes.
2. Once done, allow to release pressure naturally for 5 minutes then release remaining using quick release. Remove lid.
3. Stir well and serve.

NUTRITION:

Calories 37
Fat 0.5 g
Carbohydrates 7.4 g
Sugar 0.9 g
Protein 2 g
Cholesterol 0 mg

49. TOMATO DILL CAULIFLOWER

Preparation Time: 10 minutes

Cooking Time: 12 minutes

Servings: 4

INGREDIENTS

- 1 lb cauliflower florets, chopped
- 1 tbsp fresh dill, chopped
- 1/4 tsp Italian seasoning
- 1 tbsp vinegar
- 1 cup can tomatoes, crushed
- 1 cup vegetable stock
- 1 tsp garlic, minced
- Pepper
- Salt

DIRECTIONS

1. Seal pot with lid and cook on high for 12 minutes.
2. Once done, allow to release pressure naturally for 10 minutes then release remaining using quick release. Remove lid.
3. Garnish with dill and serve.

NUTRITION:

Calories 47

Fat 0.3 g

Carbohydrates 10 g

Sugar 5 g

Protein 3.1 g

Cholesterol 0 mg

50. PARSNIPS WITH EGGPLANT

Preparation Time: 10 minutes

Cooking Time: 12 minutes

Servings: 4

INGREDIENTS

- 2 parsnips, sliced
- 1 cup can tomatoes, crushed
- 1/2 tsp ground cumin
- 1 tbsp paprika
- 1 tsp garlic, minced
- 1 eggplant, cut into chunks
- 1/4 tsp dried basil
- Pepper
- Salt

DIRECTIONS

1. Add all ingredients into the instant pot and stir well.
2. Seal pot with lid and cook on high for 12 minutes.
3. Once done, release pressure using quick release. Remove lid.
4. Stir and serve.

NUTRITION:

Calories 98 0.7 g
Carbohydrates 23 g
Sugar 8.8 g
Protein 2.8 g
Cholesterol 0 mg

CHAPTER 12

POULTRY

51. DUCK AND BLACKBERRIES

Preparation time: 10 minutes

Cooking time: 25 minutes

Servings: 4

INGREDIENTS

- 4 duck breasts, boneless and skin scored
- 2 tablespoons balsamic vinegar
- Salt and black pepper to the taste
- 1 cup chicken stock
- 4 ounces blackberries
- ¼ cup chicken stock
- 2 tablespoons avocado oil

DIRECTIONS

1. between plates and serve.

NUTRITION:

**Calories 239,
fat 10.5,
fiber 10.2,
carbs 21.1,
protein 33.3**

52. GINGER DUCATED

Preparation time: 10 minutes

Cooking time: 50 minutes

Servings: 4

INGREDIENTS

- 2 big duck breasts, boneless and skin scored
- 2 tablespoons olive oil
- Salt and black pepper to the taste
- 1 tablespoon fish sauce
- 1 tablespoon lime juice
- 1 garlic clove, minced
- 1 Serrano chili, chopped
- 1 small shallot, sliced
- 1 cucumber, sliced
- 2 mangos, peeled and sliced
- ¼ cup oregano, chopped

DIRECTIONS

1. Heat up a pan with the oil over medium-high heat, add the duck breasts skin side down and cook for 5 minutes.
2. Add the orange zest, salt, pepper, fish sauce and the rest of the ingredients, bring to a simmer and cook over medium-low heat for 45 minutes.
3. Divide everything between plates and serve.

NUTRITION:

Calories 297,
fat 9.1,
fiber 10.2,

carbs 20.8,
protein 16.5

53. TURKEY AND CRANBERRY SAUCE

Preparation time: 10 minutes

Cooking time: 50 minutes

Servings: 4

INGREDIENTS

- 1 cup chicken stock
- 2 tablespoons avocado oil
- ½ cup cranberry sauce
- 1 big turkey breast, skinless, boneless and sliced
- 1 yellow onion, roughly chopped
- Salt and black pepper to the taste

DIRECTIONS

1. Heat up a pan with the avocado oil over medium-high heat, add the onion and sauté for 5 minutes.
2. Add the turkey and brown for 5 minutes more.
3. Add the rest of the ingredients, toss, introduce in the oven at 350 degrees F and cook for 40 minutes

NUTRITION:

Calories 382,

fat 12.6,

fiber 9.6,

carbs 26.6,

protein 17.6

54. SAGE TURKEY MIX

Preparation time: 10 minutes

Cooking time: 40 minutes

Servings: 4

INGREDIENTS

- 1 big turkey breast, skinless, boneless and roughly cubed
- Juice of 1 lemon
- 2 tablespoons avocado oil
- 1 red onion, chopped
- 2 tablespoons sage, chopped
- 1 garlic clove, minced
- 1 cup chicken stock

DIRECTIONS

1. Heat up a pan with the avocado oil over medium-high heat, add the turkey and brown for 3 minutes on each side.
2. Add the rest of the ingredients, bring to a simmer and cook over medium heat for 35 minutes.
3. Divide the mix between plates and serve with a side dish.

NUTRITION:

Calories 382,
fat 12.6,
fiber 9.6,
carbs 16.6,
protein 33.2

55. TURKEY AND ASPARAGUS MIX

Preparation time: 10 minutes

Cooking time: 30 minutes

Servings: 4

INGREDIENTS

- 1 bunch asparagus, trimmed and halved
- 1 big turkey breast, skinless, boneless and cut into strips
- 1 teaspoon basil, dried
- 2 tablespoons olive oil
- A pinch of salt and black pepper
- ½ cup tomato sauce
- 1 tablespoon chives, chopped

DIRECTIONS

1. Heat up a pan with the oil over medium-high heat, add the turkey and brown for 4 minutes.
2. Add the asparagus and the rest of the ingredients except the chives, bring to a simmer and cook over medium heat for 25 minutes.
3. Add the chives, divide the mix between plates and serve.

NUTRITION:

Calories 337,
fat 21.2,
fiber 10.2,
carbs 21.4,
protein 17.6

56. HERBED ALMOND TURKEY

Preparation time: 10 minutes

Cooking time: 40 minutes

Servings: 4

INGREDIENTS

- 1 big turkey breast, skinless, boneless and cubed
- 1 tablespoon olive oil
- ½ cup chicken stock
- 1 tablespoon basil, chopped
- 1 tablespoon rosemary, chopped
- 1 tablespoon oregano, chopped
- 1 tablespoon parsley, chopped
- 3 garlic cloves, minced
- ½ cup almonds, toasted and chopped
- 3 cups tomatoes, chopped

DIRECTIONS

1. Heat up a pan with the oil over medium-high heat, add the turkey and the garlic and brown for 5 minutes.
2. Add the stock and the rest of the ingredients, bring to a simmer over medium heat and cook for 35 minutes.
3. Divide the mix between plates and serve.

NUTRITION:

Calories 297,

fat 11.2,

fiber 9.2,

carbs 19.4,

protein 23.6

57. THYME CHICKEN AND POTATOES

Preparation time: 10 minutes

Cooking time: 50 minutes

Servings: 4

INGREDIENTS

- 1 tablespoon olive oil
- 4 garlic cloves, minced
- A pinch of salt and black pepper
- 2 teaspoons thyme, dried
- 12 small red potatoes, halved
- 2 pounds chicken breast, skinless, boneless and cubed
- 1 cup red onion, sliced
- ¾ cup chicken stock
- 2 tablespoons basil, chopped

DIRECTIONS

1. In a baking dish greased with the oil, add the potatoes, chicken and the rest of the ingredients, toss a bit, introduce in the oven and bake at 400 degrees F for 50 minutes.
2. Divide between plates and serve.

NUTRITION:

Calories 281,
fat 9.2,
fiber 10.9,
carbs 21.6,
protein 13.6

58. TURKEY, ARTICHOKES AND ASPARAGUS

Preparation time: 10 minutes

Cooking time: 30 minutes

Servings: 4

INGREDIENTS

- 2 turkey breasts, boneless, skinless and halved
- 3 tablespoons olive oil
- 1 and ½ pounds asparagus, trimmed and halved
- 1 cup chicken stock
- A pinch of salt and black pepper
- 1 cup canned artichoke hearts, drained
- ¼ cup kalamata olives, pitted and sliced
- 1 shallot, chopped
- 3 garlic cloves, minced
- 3 tablespoons dill, chopped

DIRECTIONS

1. Heat up a pan with the oil over medium-high heat, add the turkey and the garlic and brown for 4 minutes on each side.
2. Add the asparagus, the stock and the rest of the ingredients except the dill, bring to a simmer and cook over medium heat for 20 minutes.
3. Add the dill, divide the mix between plates and serve.

NUTRITION:

Calories 291,
fat 16,
fiber 10.3,

carbs 22.8,
protein 34.5

59. LEMONY TURKEY AND PINE NUTS

Preparation time: 10 minutes

Cooking time: 30 minutes

Servings: 4

INGREDIENTS

- 2 turkey breasts, boneless, skinless and halved
- A pinch of salt and black pepper
- 2 tablespoons avocado oil
- Juice of 2 lemons
- 1 tablespoon rosemary, chopped
- 3 garlic cloves, minced
- ¼ cup pine nuts, chopped
- 1 cup chicken stock

DIRECTIONS

1. Heat up a pan with the oil over medium-high heat, add the garlic and the turkey and brown for 4 minutes on each side.
2. Add the rest of the ingredients, bring to a simmer and cook over medium heat for 20 minutes.
3. Divide the mix between plates and serve with a side salad.

NUTRITION:

Calories 293,
fat 12.4,
fiber 9.3,
carbs 17.8,
protein 24.5

60. YOGURT CHICKEN AND RED ONION MIX

Preparation time: 10 minutes

Cooking time: 30 minutes

Servings: 4

INGREDIENTS

- 2 pounds chicken breast, skinless, boneless and sliced
- 3 tablespoons olive oil
- ¼ cup Greek yogurt
- 2 garlic cloves, minced
- ½ teaspoon onion powder
- A pinch of salt and black pepper
- 4 red onions, sliced

DIRECTIONS

1. In a roasting pan, combine the chicken with the oil, the yogurt and the other ingredients, introduce in the oven at 375 degrees F and bake for 30 minutes.
2. Divide chicken mix between plates and serve hot.

NUTRITION:

Calories 278,
fat 15,
fiber 9.2,
carbs 15.1,
protein 23.3

CHAPTER 13

MEAT

61. MOIST SHREDDED BEEF

Preparation Time: 10 minutes

Cooking Time: 20 minutes

Servings: 8

INGREDIENTS

- 2 lbs beef chuck roast, cut into chunks
- 1/2 tbsp dried red pepper
- 1 tbsp Italian seasoning
- 1 tbsp garlic, minced
- 2 tbsp vinegar
- 14 oz can fire-roasted tomatoes
- 1/2 cup bell pepper, chopped
- 1/2 cup carrots, chopped
- 1 cup onion, chopped
- 1 tsp salt

DIRECTIONS

1. Add all ingredients into the inner pot of instant pot and set the pot on sauté mode.
2. Seal pot with lid and cook on high for 20 minutes.
3. Once done, release pressure using quick release. Remove lid.
4. Shred the meat using a fork.
5. Stir well and serve.

NUTRITION:

Calories 456
Fat 32.7 g
Carbohydrates 7.7 g
Sugar 4.1 g
Protein 31 g
Cholesterol 118 mg

62. HEARTY BEEF RAGU

Preparation Time: 10 minutes

Cooking Time: 50 minutes

Servings: 4

INGREDIENTS

- 1 1/2 lbs beef steak, diced
- 1 1/2 cup beef stock
- 1 tbsp coconut amino
- 14 oz can tomatoes, chopped
- 1/2 tsp ground cinnamon
- 1 tsp dried thyme
- 1 tsp dried basil
- 1 tsp paprika
- 1 bay leaf
- 1 tbsp garlic, chopped
- 1/2 tsp cayenne pepper
- 1 celery stick, diced
- 1 carrot, diced
- 1 onion, diced
- 2 tbsp olive oil
- 1/4 tsp pepper
- 1 1/2 tsp sea salt

DIRECTIONS

1. Add oil into the instant pot and set the pot on sauté mode.
2. Add celery, carrots, onion, and salt and sauté for 5 minutes.
3. Add meat and remaining ingredients and stir everything well.

4.   Seal pot with lid and cook on high for 30 minutes.
5.   Once done, allow to release pressure naturally for 10 minutes then release remaining using quick release. Remove lid.
6.   Shred meat using a fork. Set pot on sauté mode and cook for 10 minutes. Stir every 2-3 minutes.
7.   Serve and enjoy.

NUTRITION:

Calories 435
Fat 18.1 g
Carbohydrates 12.3 g
Sugar 5.5 g
Protein 54.4 g
Cholesterol 152 mg

63. DILL BEEF BRISKET

Preparation Time: 10 minutes

Cooking Time: 50 minutes

Servings: 4

INGREDIENTS

- 2 1/2 lbs beef brisket, cut into cubes
- 2 1/2 cups beef stock
- 2 tbsp dill, chopped
- 1 celery stalk, chopped
- 1 onion, sliced
- 1 tbsp garlic, minced
- Pepper
- Salt

DIRECTIONS

1. Add all ingredients into the inner pot of instant pot and stir well.
2. Seal pot with lid and cook on high for 50 minutes.
3. Once done, allow to release pressure naturally for 10 minutes then release remaining using quick release. Remove lid.
4. Serve and enjoy.

NUTRITION:

Calories 556

Fat 18.1 g

Carbohydrates 4.3 g

Sugar 1.3 g

Protein 88.5 g

Cholesterol 253 mg

64. TASTY BEEF STEW

Preparation Time: 10 minutes

Cooking Time: 30 minutes

Servings: 4

INGREDIENTS

- 2 1/2 lbs beef roast, cut into chunks
- 1 cup beef broth
- 1/2 cup balsamic vinegar
- 1 tbsp honey
- 1/2 tsp red pepper flakes
- 1 tbsp garlic, minced
- Pepper
- Salt

DIRECTIONS

1. Add all ingredients into the inner pot of instant pot and stir well.
2. Seal pot with lid and cook on high for 30 minutes.
3. Once done, allow to release pressure naturally. Remove lid.
4. Stir well and serve.

NUTRITION:

Calories 562

Fat 18.1 g

Carbohydrates 5.7 g

Sugar 4.6 g

Protein 87.4 g

Cholesterol 253 mg

65. MEATLOAF

Preparation Time: 10 minutes

Cooking Time: 35 minutes

Servings: 6

INGREDIENTS

- 2 lbs ground beef
- 2 eggs, lightly beaten
- 1/4 tsp dried basil
- 3 tbsp olive oil
- 1/2 tsp dried sage
- 1 1/2 tsp dried parsley
- 1 tsp oregano
- 2 tsp thyme
- 1 tsp rosemary
- Pepper
- Salt

DIRECTIONS

1. Pour 1 1/2 cups of water into the instant pot then place the trivet in the pot.
2. Spray loaf pan with cooking spray.
3. Add all ingredients into the mixing bowl and mix until well combined.
4. Transfer meat mixture into the prepared loaf pan and place loaf pan on top of the trivet in the pot.
5. Seal pot with lid and cook on high for 35 minutes.

6. Once done, allow to release pressure naturally for 10 minutes then release remaining using quick release. Remove lid.
7. Serve and enjoy.

NUTRITION:

Calories 365
Fat 18 g
Carbohydrates 0.7 g
Sugar 0.1 g
Protein 47.8 g
Cholesterol 190 mg

66. FLAVORFUL BEEF BOURGUIGNON

Preparation Time: 10 minutes

Cooking Time: 20 minutes

Servings: 4

INGREDIENTS

- 1 1/2 lbs beef chuck roast, cut into chunks
- 2/3 cup beef stock
- 2 tbsp fresh thyme
- 1 bay leaf
- 1 tsp garlic, minced
- 8 oz mushrooms, sliced
- 2 tbsp tomato paste
- 2/3 cup dry red wine
- 1 onion, sliced
- 4 carrots, cut into chunks
- 1 tbsp olive oil
- Pepper
- Salt

DIRECTIONS

1. Add oil into the instant pot and set the pot on sauté mode.
2. Add meat and sauté until brown. Add onion and sauté until softened.
3. Add remaining ingredients and stir well.
4. Seal pot with lid and cook on high for 12 minutes.
5. Once done, allow to release pressure naturally. Remove lid.
6. Stir well and serve.

NUTRITION:

Calories 744

Fat 51.3 g

Carbohydrates 14.5 g

Sugar 6.5 g

Protein 48.1 g

Cholesterol 175 mg

67. DELICIOUS BEEF CHILI

Preparation Time: 10 minutes

Cooking Time: 35 minutes

Servings: 8

INGREDIENTS

- 2 lbs ground beef
- 1 tsp olive oil
- 1 tsp garlic, minced
- 1 small onion, chopped
- 2 tbsp chili powder
- 1 tsp oregano
- 1/2 tsp thyme
- 28 oz can tomatoes, crushed
- 2 cups beef stock
- 2 carrots, chopped
- 3 sweet potatoes, peeled and cubed
- Pepper
- Salt

DIRECTIONS

1. Add oil into the instant pot and set the pot on sauté mode.
2. Add meat and cook until brown.
3. Add remaining ingredients and stir well.
4. Seal pot with lid and cook on high for 35 minutes.
5. Once done, allow to release pressure naturally. Remove lid.
6. Stir well and serve.

NUTRITION:

Calories 302

Fat 8.2 g

Carbohydrates 19.2 g

Sugar 4.8 g

Protein 37.1 g

Cholesterol 101 mg

68. ROSEMARY CREAMY BEEF

Preparation Time: 10 minutes

Cooking Time: 40 minutes

Servings: 4

INGREDIENTS

- 2 lbs beef stew meat, cubed
- 2 tbsp fresh parsley, chopped
- 1 tsp garlic, minced
- 1/2 tsp dried rosemary
- 1 tsp chili powder
- 1 cup beef stock
- 1 cup heavy cream
- 1 onion, chopped
- 1 tbsp olive oil
- Pepper
- Salt

DIRECTIONS

1. Add oil into the instant pot and set the pot on sauté mode.
2. Add rosemary, garlic, onion, and chili powder and sauté for 5 minutes.
3. Add meat and cook for 5 minutes.
4. Add remaining ingredients and stir well.
5. Seal pot with lid and cook on high for 30 minutes.

6. Once done, allow to release pressure naturally for 10 minutes then release remaining using quick release. Remove lid.
7. Serve and enjoy.

NUTRITION:

Calories 574
Fat 29 g
Carbohydrates 4.3 g
Sugar 1.3 g
Protein 70.6 g
Cholesterol 244 mg

69. SPICY BEEF CHILI VERDE

Preparation Time: 10 minutes

Cooking Time: 23 minutes

Servings: 2

INGREDIENTS

- 1/2 lb beef stew meat, cut into cubes
- 1/4 tsp chili powder
- 1 tbsp olive oil
- 1 cup chicken broth
- 1 Serrano pepper, chopped
- 1 tsp garlic, minced
- 1 small onion, chopped
- 1/4 cup grape tomatoes, chopped
- 1/4 cup tomatillos, chopped
- Pepper
- Salt

DIRECTIONS

1. Add oil into the instant pot and set the pot on sauté mode.
2. Add garlic and onion and sauté for 3 minutes.
3. Add remaining ingredients and stir well.
4. Seal pot with lid and cook on high for 20 minutes.
5. Once done, allow to release pressure naturally. Remove lid.
6. Stir well and serve.

NUTRITION:

Calories 317

Fat 15.1 g

Carbohydrates 6.4 g

Sugar 2.6 g

Protein 37.8 g

Cholesterol 101 mg

70. CARROT MUSHROOM BEEF ROAST

Preparation Time: 10 minutes

Cooking Time: 40 minutes

Servings: 4

INGREDIENTS

- 1 1/2 lbs beef roast
- 1 tsp paprika
- 1/4 tsp dried rosemary
- 1 tsp garlic, minced
- 1/2 lb mushrooms, sliced
- 1/2 cup chicken stock
- 2 carrots, sliced
- Pepper
- Salt

DIRECTIONS

1. Add all ingredients into the inner pot of instant pot and stir well.
2. Seal pot with lid and cook on high for 40 minutes.
3. Once done, allow to release pressure naturally for 10 minutes then release remaining using quick release. Remove lid.
4. Slice and serve.

NUTRITION:

Calories 345

Fat 10.9 g

Carbohydrates 5.6 g

Sugar 2.6 g

Protein 53.8 g

Cholesterol 152 mg

CHAPTER 14

SNACKS

71. GARLIC PINTO BEAN DIP

Preparation Time: 10 minutes

Cooking Time: 43 minutes

Servings: 6

INGREDIENTS

- 1 cup dry pinto beans, rinsed
- 1/2 tsp cumin
- 1/2 cup salsa
- 2 garlic cloves
- 2 chipotle peppers in adobo sauce
- 5 cups vegetable stock
- Pepper
- Salt

DIRECTIONS

1. Add beans, stock, garlic, and chipotle peppers into the instant pot.
2. Seal pot with lid and cook on high for 43 minutes.
3. Once done, release pressure using quick release. Remove lid.
4. Drain beans well and reserve 1/2 cup of stock.
5. Transfer beans, reserve stock, and remaining ingredients into the food processor and process until smooth.
6. Serve and enjoy.

NUTRITION:

Calories 129
Fat 0.9 g
Carbohydrates 23 g
Sugar 1.9 g
Protein 8 g
Cholesterol 2 mg

72. CREAMY EGGPLANT DIP

Preparation Time: 10 minutes

Cooking Time: 20 minutes

Servings: 4

INGREDIENTS

- 1 eggplant
- 1/2 tsp paprika
- 1 tbsp olive oil
- 1 tbsp fresh lime juice
- 2 tbsp tahini
- 1 garlic clove
- 1 cup of water
- Pepper
- Salt

DIRECTIONS

1. Add water and eggplant into the instant pot.
2. Seal pot with the lid and select manual and set timer for 20 minutes.
3. Once done, release pressure using quick release. Remove lid.
4. Drain eggplant and let it cool.
5. Once the eggplant is cool then remove eggplant skin and transfer eggplant flesh into the food processor.
6. Add remaining ingredients into the food processor and process until smooth.
7. Serve and enjoy.

NUTRITION:

Calories 108

Fat 7.8 g

Carbohydrates 9.7 g

Sugar 3.7 g

Protein 2.5 g

Cholesterol 0 mg

73. JALAPENO CHICKPEA HUMMUS

Preparation Time: 10 minutes

Cooking Time: 25 minutes

Servings: 4

INGREDIENTS

- 1 cup dry chickpeas, soaked overnight and drained
- 1 tsp ground cumin
- 1/4 cup jalapenos, diced
- 1/2 cup fresh cilantro
- 1 tbsp tahini
- 1/2 cup olive oil
- Pepper
- Salt

DIRECTIONS

1. Add chickpeas into the instant pot and cover with vegetable stock.
2. Seal pot with lid and cook on high for 25 minutes.
3. Once done, allow to release pressure naturally. Remove lid.
4. Drain chickpeas well and transfer into the food processor along with remaining ingredients and process until smooth.
5. Serve and enjoy.

NUTRITION:

Calories 425

Fat 30.4 g

Carbohydrates 31.8 g

Sugar 5.6 g

Protein 10.5 g

Cholesterol 0 mg

74. TASTY BLACK BEAN DIP

Preparation Time: 10 minutes

Cooking Time: 18 minutes

Servings: 6

INGREDIENTS

- 2 cups dry black beans, soaked overnight and drained
- 1 1/2 cups cheese, shredded
- 1 tsp dried oregano
- 1 1/2 tsp chili powder
- 2 cups tomatoes, chopped
- 2 tbsp olive oil
- 1 1/2 tbsp garlic, minced
- 1 medium onion, sliced
- 4 cups vegetable stock
- Pepper
- Salt

DIRECTIONS

1. Add all ingredients except cheese into the instant pot.
2. Seal pot with lid and cook on high for 18 minutes.
3. Once done, allow to release pressure naturally. Remove lid. Drain excess water.
4. Add cheese and stir until cheese is melted.
5. Blend bean mixture using an immersion blender until smooth.
6. Serve and enjoy.

NUTRITION:

Calories 402
Fat 15.3 g
Carbohydrates 46.6 g

Sugar 4.4 g
Protein 22.2 g
Cholesterol 30 mg

75. HEALTHY KIDNEY BEAN DIP

Preparation Time: 10 minutes

Cooking Time: 10 minutes

Servings: 6

INGREDIENTS

- 1 cup dry white kidney beans, soaked overnight and drained
- 1 tbsp fresh lemon juice
- 2 tbsp water
- 1/2 cup coconut yogurt
- 1 roasted garlic clove
- 1 tbsp olive oil
- 1/4 tsp cayenne
- 1 tsp dried parsley
- Pepper
- Salt

DIRECTIONS

1. Add soaked beans and 1 3/4 cups of water into the instant pot.
2. Seal pot with lid and cook on high for 10 minutes.
3. Once done, allow to release pressure naturally. Remove lid.
4. Drain beans well and transfer them into the food processor.
5. Add remaining ingredients into the food processor and process until smooth.
6. Serve and enjoy.

NUTRITION:

Calories 136

Fat 3.2 g

Carbohydrates 20 g

Sugar 2.1 g

Protein 7.7 g

Cholesterol 0 mg

CHAPTER 15

DESSERTS & FRUIT

76. VANILLA APPLE COMPOTE

Preparation Time: 10 minutes

Cooking Time: 15 minutes

Servings: 6

INGREDIENTS

- 3 cups apples, cored and cubed
- 1 tsp vanilla
- 3/4 cup coconut sugar
- 1 cup of water
- 2 tbsp fresh lime juice

DIRECTIONS

1. Seal pot with lid and cook on high for 15 minutes.
2. Once done, allow to release pressure naturally for 10 minutes then release remaining using quick release. Remove lid.
3. Stir and serve.

NUTRITION:

Calories 76
Fat 0.2 g
Carbohydrates 19.1 g
Sugar 11.9 g
Protein 0.5 g
Cholesterol 0 mg

77. APPLE DATES MIX

Preparation Time: 10 minutes

Cooking Time: 15 minutes

Servings: 4

INGREDIENTS

- 4 apples, cored and cut into chunks
- 1 tsp vanilla
- 1 tsp cinnamon
- 1/2 cup dates, pitted
- 1 1/2 cups apple juice

DIRECTIONS

1. Seal pot with lid and cook on high for 15 minutes.
2. Once done, allow to release pressure naturally for 10 minutes then release remaining using quick release. Remove lid.
3. Stir and serve.

NUTRITION:

Calories 226
Fat 0.6 g
Carbohydrates 58.6 g
Sugar 46.4 g
Protein 1.3 g
Cholesterol 0 mg

78. CHOCO RICE PUDDING

Preparation Time: 10 minutes

Cooking Time: 20 minutes

Servings: 4

INGREDIENTS

- 1 1/4 cup rice
- 1/4 cup dark chocolate, chopped
- 1 tsp vanilla
- 1/3 cup coconut butter
- 1 tsp liquid stevia
- 2 1/2 cups almond milk

DIRECTIONS

1. Seal pot with lid and cook on high for 20 minutes.
2. Once done, allow to release pressure naturally. Remove lid.
3. Stir well and serve.

NUTRITION:

Calories 632
Fat 39.9 g
Carbohydrates 63.5 g
Sugar 12.5 g
Protein 8.6 g
Cholesterol 2 mg

79. GRAPES STEW

Preparation Time: 10 minutes

Cooking Time: 15 minutes

Servings: 4

INGREDIENTS

- 1 cup grapes, halved
- 1 tsp vanilla
- 1 tbsp fresh lemon juice
- 1 tbsp honey
- 2 cups rhubarb, chopped
- 2 cups of water

DIRECTIONS

1. Seal pot with lid and cook on high for 15 minutes.
2. Once done, allow to release pressure naturally for 10 minutes then release remaining using quick release. Remove lid.
3. Stir and serve.

NUTRITION:

Calories 48
Fat 0.2 g
Carbohydrates 11.3 g
Sugar 8.9 g
Protein 0.7 g
Cholesterol 0 mg

80. CHOCOLATE RICE

Preparation Time: 10 minutes

Cooking Time: 20 minutes

Servings: 4

INGREDIENTS

- 1 cup of rice
- 1 tbsp cocoa powder
- 2 tbsp maple syrup
- 2 cups almond milk

DIRECTIONS

1. Add all ingredients into the inner pot of instant pot and stir well.
2. Seal pot with lid and cook on high for 20 minutes.
3. Once done, allow to release pressure naturally for 10 minutes then release remaining using quick release. Remove lid.
4. Stir and serve.

NUTRITION:

Calories 474
Fat 29.1 g
Carbohydrates 51.1 g
Sugar 10 g
Protein 6.3 g
Cholesterol 0 mg

CONCLUSION

The Mediterranean diet is more than what you eat; it is a way of living. This diet reflects the true definition of what a diet should be. It encourages eating healthy nutritious foods, while also emphasizing the importance of physical activity and spending time with those we care about. The Mediterranean diet has been studied for decades and each time it seems a new benefit of this diet comes to light.

Although there are studies that back up the benefits of the Mediterranean diet, and although it has been reviewed countless times and tested on various individuals with varying complications, it has yet to be the standard way of living around the world.

What needs to be done is adopting a new way of looking at food and mealtimes. Our world today stresses working harder and longer which means there is little time for enjoying meals. If we can change our perspective to see that the food we eat is what makes us more efficient and productive, then we would be able to change the way we eat more efficiently.

The Mediterranean diet considers various aspects of what "health" means. It does not just focus on what you eat but it also focuses on how you eat, who you eat with, and the activities you do in between eating. Each of these components can contribute to better health and a more fulfilling life. When we are lacking in any of these components, we tend to suffer from poor health, fatigue, depression and more. The

Mediterranean diet was initially looked at because of its heart health benefits, but now it is clear to see that the traditional Mediterranean lifestyle from the 1950s was more than just a heart-healthy plan.

The changes can be made in small steps, because even the slightest change to shifting your diet to a more Mediterranean diet can have a whirlwind of benefits. You have learned how to swap the unhealthy foods you have been used to consuming with nutrient-dense and wholesome foods.

You now have a better understanding that this diet is not about just losing weight. It is not a diet that allows you to eat your weight in pasta, or drink equal amounts of red wine. It has shown that you can use food as a form of natural medicine to reduce and eliminate the risk of many severe health conditions. You have learned how your food directly affects the way your body functions and when it is deprived of the nutrients it needs it will not be able to perform appropriately.

Now that you have all this information on how you can maintain and achieve optimal health, it is up to you to decide. Will you continue to choose a life where the foods you eat leads you down a road to illness and preventable suffering? Or will you make the change now to live your life and be the healthiest and happiest version of you? All you have to do is start with one small change and then go from there. Once you begin to see the benefits from that one little choice you will be eager to try more and soon you will be living a Mediterranean lifestyle that is significantly more satisfying.